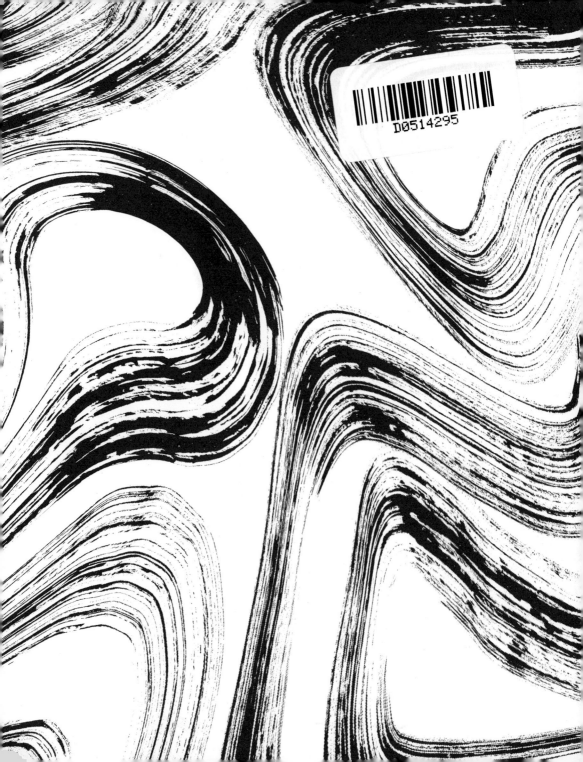

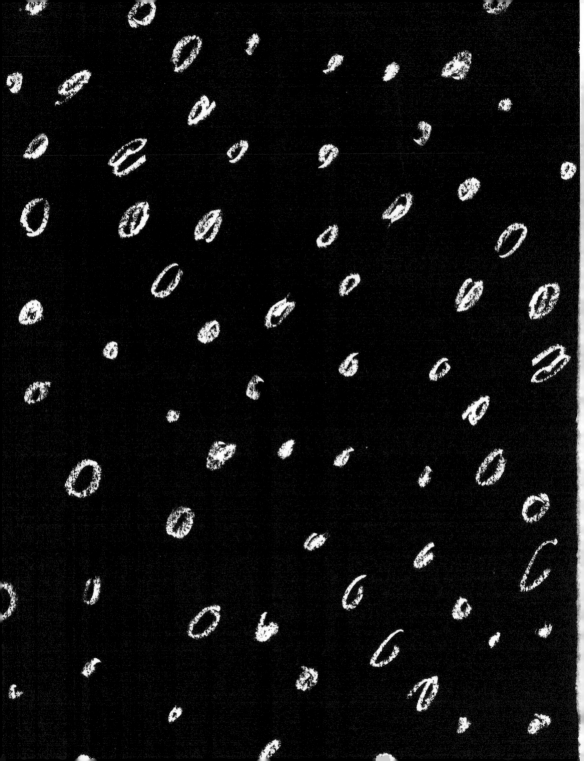

## FIVE

*Beauty thingies the author could live without, but would really prefer not to.*

**One**
A moisturising physical sunscreen with broad-spectrum SPF30 protection for daily wear, cos she is no goose.

**Two**
Dry shampoo applied on clean, fluffy hair for perceived dirtiness, and on filthy hair for perceived cleanliness.

**Three**
An anti-inflammatory, antioxidant-crammed face oil to juice up the skin and defend it from all them dang aggressors.

**Four**
A glossy, nourishing lip balm that can also rapidly plump up fine lines around the eyes or soothe angry cuticles if things get desperate.

**Five**
A professional hair and makeup artist living in a granny flat out back.

Also by Zoë Foster (Blake)

**Air Kisses**

**Playing the Field**

**The Younger Man**

**The Wrong Girl**
(This one was made into a telly show!)

**Textbook Romance**
(with Hamish Blake)

**Amazing Face**
(Oh come on, it counts, surely.)

Fully revised and updated!
Over 60 new pages!
New longer title!

# amazinger

# FACE

## ZOË FOSTER (Blake)

CLEVER BEAUTY TRICKS,
SHOULD-OWN PRODUCTS,
SPECTACULARLY USEFUL
HOW-TO-DO-ITS

VIKING
*an imprint of*
PENGUIN BOOKS

VIKING

UK | USA | Canada | Ireland | Australia
India | New Zealand | South Africa | China

Penguin Books is part of the Penguin Random House group of companies
whose addresses can be found at global.penguinrandomhouse.com.

First published by Penguin Group (Australia), 2011
This revised edition published by Penguin Group (Australia), 2016

Design and illustration by Allison Colpoys
Illustration of Go-To Face Hero on page IX by Alice Oehr
Photographs by Tim de Neefe
Hair and makeup by Belinda Zollo
Floral neckpiece on page 283 by Ann Shoebridge: annshoebridge.com
Colour reproduction by Splitting Image Pty Ltd, Clayton, Victoria
Printed and bound in China by 1010 Printing International Limited

National Library of Australia
Cataloguing-in-Publication data:

Foster, Zoë.
Amazinger face / Zoë Foster.
9780670078233 (pbk.)
Includes index.
Beauty, Personal.
Cosmetics.

646.7042

penguin.com.au

# CONTENTS:

This page has been scented with an exquisite medley of exotic, cold-pressed paper, Bulgarian ink extract and sparkling, fruity words to further enhance your sensory enjoyment of reading Amazinger Face. Please enjoy.

# INTRODUCTION:

## I learned how to apply makeup from a girl in the school toilets.

She was an exquisite, popular, sophisticated* year nine girl (I was a year eight dork and the girls in the year above were deities for reasons I can only put down to 'having pashed boys already'), and it was spellbinding to see her face transform.

Sadly, my facsimile was not the flawless masterpiece I'd hoped for, although I *was* able to generously offer my family several solid hours of amusement.

*But what the heck was a girl to do?* My options were my older sister, who was noisily stomping through her punk stage and wildly unhelpful, my mum, who wore nothing but Anais Anais and lipstick, or my friends, who were still hypnotised by Lip Smackers and unwilling to progress. The Girl in the School Toilets was my best chance.

Astonishingly, learning makeup application from a Girl in the School Toilets (who invariably learned it from someone equally as unqualified) is not as valuable as one might think.

But I persisted, experimenting with beauty in all its forms through the tragicomedy of high school with the application technique of a drunken bat. Eye shadow? Whatever shade is on sale at the chemist! Hair colour? Whichever colour looks most fun! Skin care? Whatever mum buys me! Screw technique, sugar; *just get it on there!* Oh, and whatever you do, PLUCK YOUR EYEBROWS. Pluck them a lot. Have no idea why or

*It's all relative.*

how, just do it because everyone else is. See? See how pretty they look all thin and wonky and uneven like that? Great job!

This spectacular incompetence continued until I was 23, when I became beauty editor at *Cosmopolitan*. To this day no one is sure how. My only eye shadow at that time was a frosty green CoverGirl one, and you bet your bronzer I wore it to the interview.

Two days in and I was interviewing the gent responsible for cutting Jennifer Aniston's hair, and so my on-job learning commenced.

People mistakenly think beauty editors are makeup artists or beauty therapists turned writers, but we are not. Those guys are incredibly knowledgeable in one area, whereas we know lots of little things about many areas. The goal is to inhale as much info as possible on everything beauty-related, from every available source, then elegantly spit it out in an accessible fashion for our readers.

And for over a decade, I did. Every time I interviewed a hair or makeup artist, I learned exciting new tricks that changed the way I did my own hair and face. Ditto with the dermatologists and scientists I met along the way. *These people know their shit*. They are the finest in their field! Beauty is their passion and their profession! God bless them and their smarts and trickery!

My fellow beauty editors were also tremendously inspiring: you cannot imagine such a glorious constellation of stylish, mischievous, talented dames! Intimidatingly proficient with any beauty tool or product in their orbit, and magnificent at sassing a trend before it even knows it's a trend. Shimmering peacock-green liner and a frisky new fringe here, melon lips and duck-egg blue toenails over there...Being a beauty editor is a circus of invention and playfulness, and I hurled myself into it with zest and jubilance. So much so that in 2006 I felt compelled to start a beauty blog in addition to working full-time as a beauty editor. GREAT SQUIDS OF MADRID WAS I PASSIONATE ABOUT LIP LINER AND SHAMPOO.

I'm no longer an active beauty editor. Since the first edition of this book was published in 2011, things have changed (like products, for example, which is why I have updated them in this new edition), largely because of feedback I had from you guys. You insisted I drop this beauty palaver to become an astrophysicist, and finally I am. Just kidding! Too easy. I like a challenge. So I created my own skin care range, Go-To, instead.

I did this because there are only three billion skin care products out there and obviously more were needed. Also, I knew how frustrated and confused you guys were by face creams and exfoliators and serums. And understandably so! Skin care is a tricky, rapidly changing puzzle. So, I jammed all the education I had on the topic plus all of the ingredients I knew to be effective into an all-natural, tight edit of essentials, and launched it. It's good stuff and I'm very proud of it, and Mum says it's nice so it must be. You'll see it mentioned a *few* times within these pages (don't worry, I haven't been vulgar about it, and just ignore that skywriter up above, I'm pretty sure he's writing *Bo-To*) because when you create a cleanser that combines all the things you want and need in a cleanser, it feels somehow disingenuous recommending another brand or type.

But who gives a turtle's toot! It's time for you sweet peanuts to gallop squealing into *Amazinger Face*! A book that will make you feel competent and confident with beauty, and prove that it *isn't* intimidating or confusing, but rather enjoyable, easy and exciting.

Learn (or re-learn) the basics, and master some new stuff. Take what works for you and chuck what doesn't. Challenge what you've always done or thought. Play. Nick these tips and announce them as your own, rather like I did in putting this book together, although let it be known *I would never suggest I created these tips*: they either came to me via dreams (false) or were taught to me by the best in the business over the years (true).

Enjoy it, you gorgeous rascals!

Zo x

*P. S.*

*The tips and tricks in* Amazinger Face *work for me, but may not work for everybody. I tried my best to choose the most universal, and hope you get some use from them. Also, all errors are intentional, unless unintentional.*

*PLUG!*

*Wherever the author has vulgarly mentioned her own skin care brand, Go-To, you will see this little symbol so that you know it's hers. This has been done in the interest of full transparency, and because Zoë cares about integrity and respects her readers.*

*(She was going to use a picture of a fat pig in a waistcoat smoking a cigar made of $100 notes but it seemed a bit crude. So she gave the pig some pants, and it looked much better. But then the image was too big, so she switched to the little yelly plug illustration you see at the top of these paragraphs. Perfect!)*

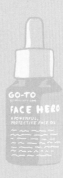

GO-TO
FACE HERO
A POWERFUL PROTECTIVE FACE OIL

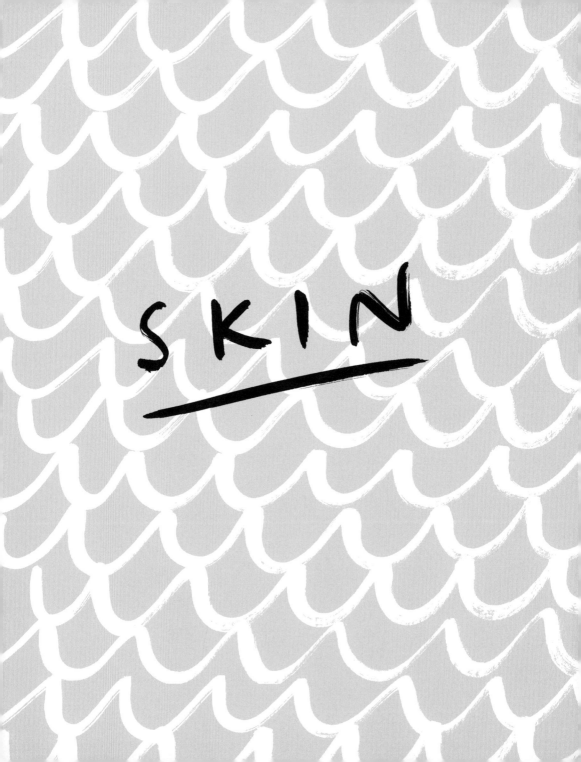

SKIN

As a wise man (probably me) once said: all the makeup and all the blow-dries and all the Céline handbags in the world don't mean much if your skin is unhappy, unsightly and uncared for.

The point: happy, healthy, radiant skin is your finest and most powerful accessory!

(Unless you're wearing a motorbike helmet, in which case it will be your handbag or belt.)

# YOUR FACE STOPS AT YOUR BOOBS.

Not at your chin or jawline or where your neck meets your décolletage. *At your boobs.*

Consider how many items in that fancy wardrobe of yours expose your chest: singlets, t-shirts, fun vintage frocks, cardigans, snazzy low-cut sexy-sexy tops – even your boring black long-sleeved top, the one you wear to the shops to get groceries, even *that hideous thing* shows off your collarbones and takes innocent bystanders halfway down to Mount Everbreast. Which is precisely why you must treat the delicate and alluring skin on the neck, collarbones and chest as you would your face.

The skin is just as thin, just as prone to wrinkles and creases and just as ripe for sun damage, and rarely will there come a time when it is not on show along with your face. *Even when you're 75.*

And even if your face has been lifted and lasered and botoxed and IPL-ed and plumped up with expensive fillers in an attempt to halt youth in her rollerblades as she cruises out the door, your neck and chest will always give away your real age.

**From today, you should totally do this:** Put whatever you put on your face in the morning and night (toner, serum, face oil, moisturiser and sun protection) on your neck and chest, too. And opt for high-necked tops and dresses as much as possible in summer. If you don't want to use your Good Face Stuff over so much surface area, then buy a second, cheaper face cream and use that instead.

**Remember:** Spending frillions on the finest creams and treatments to keep your face looking youthful means nothing if your neck-n-dec aren't given the same protection and attention.

**Q:** Which order does everything go?

**A:** In general, go from thinnest to thickest. For example, you would cleanse, then tone or clarify, then apply actives and treatment serums (which are usually liquids or gels), then face oils, then eye cream, then moisturiser with a high level of sunscreen. (Followed by primer then makeup.) (And a quick selfie cos you look cute.)

*Bonus trick!*

*Your neck ages even faster than that cute face of yours. But a specific neck product isn't required. Avoid 'turkey neck' (until you feel like getting laser skin tightening) by wearing sunscreen on the area every day, applying an antioxidant rich moisturiser that nourishes and repairs, and exfoliate with AHAs. So, um, treat it like your face, in other words.*

# HOW TO (BRIEFLY) LOOK AFTER YOUR SKIN BY AGE.

**IF YOU'RE PRE-TEEN, OR A TEENAGER**

- Start getting a basic routine together
- Use a gentle, non-drying, non-soap cleanser morning and night (and definitely remove makeup at night)
- Wear a non-oily SPF 30 each day (in addition to, or in place of, moisturiser) on face/neck/chest
- Moisturise your whole body each day after you shower

**Things to look for:**

- Salicylic acid (BHAs) or gentle AHA exfoliants
- Oil-free and non-comedogenic moisturisers and sunscreens
- Irritant-free formulas
- Clay-based masks

**IN YOUR LATE TEENS AND 20s**

- Use a gentle cleanser each morning and night (double cleanse at night, or use a makeup remover before your cleanser if you need to)
- Use antioxidants each morning to protect the skin
- Wear SPF 30 each day (in addition to, or in place of, moisturiser) on face/neck/chest
- Use an antioxidant-rich serum, face oil, and/or moisturiser (down to the boobs) each night

- Keep oil imbalances and congestion in check with regular chemical exfoliation, and, if needed, the occasional in-salon microdermabrasion or peel
- Moisturise your whole body each day after you shower

**Things to look for:**

- Antioxidants (coenzyme Q10, green tea, idebenone, resveratrol, vitamins E and C)
- AHA/BHA chemical exfoliators (glycolic/salicylic acid) for acne/breakouts
- Mineral/physical (a.k.a. zinc oxide-based or titanium dioxide) sun protection

**IN YOUR 30s**

- Use a (non-foaming/non-scrubby!) cleanser morning and night
- Use antioxidants each morning to protect the skin
- Wear SPF 30 sun protection each day (in addition to, or in place of, moisturiser) on face/neck/chest/hands
- Use an antioxidant-rich serum, face oil, and/or moisturiser (down to the boobs) each night
- Assist cell renewal and improve brightness with regular AHA-based exfoliation

- Consider an eye cream to treat dark circles/puffiness/fine lines (see page 36)
- Implement treatment serums for any specific concerns (pigmentation/acne/wrinkles)
- Consider retinol (if not pregnant/breastfeeding) for collagen production and skin renewal
- Boost hydration with nourishing face oils and hydrating masks
- Consider regular professional facials or treatments (e.g.: microdermabrasion/peels/IPL)
- Moisturise your whole body each day after you shower

**Things to look for:**
- Antioxidants (coenzyme Q10, green tea, idebenone, resveratrol, vitamins E and C)
- AHA chemical exfoliators (lactic/glycolic acid)
- Niacinamide (vitamin B3) to lighten early signs of pigmentation
- Mineral/physical (a.k.a. zinc oxide-based or titanium dioxide) sun protection
- Hyaluronic acid, glycerin, sodium PCA, plant oils and shea butter for plump, hydrated skin
- Retinol (unless pregnant or breastfeeding)

**IN YOUR 40s**
- Use a mousse/cream cleanser each morning and night
- Use antioxidants each morning to protect the skin
- Wear SPF 30 each day (in addition to, or in place of, moisturiser) on face/neck/chest/hands
- Use an antioxidant/peptide-rich, anti-ageing night cream (down to the boobs)
- Assist cell renewal and improve brightness with AHA-based exfoliation
- Consider an eye cream (see page 36)
- Use retinol to ward off wrinkles, pigmentation, etc.
- Introduce growth factors/peptide serums/creams to stimulate collagen/elastin, and support any cosmetic injectables you might choose to use
- Boost hydration with nourishing face oils and hydrating masks
- Consider professional treatments and services (e.g.: skin resurfacing, botox or laser)
- Prevent skin ageing by using plenty of moisture-rich antioxidants
- Moisturise your whole body each day after you shower

**Things to look for:**

- Antioxidants (coenzyme Q10, green tea idebenone, resveratrol, vitamins E and C)
- AHA chemical exfoliators (lactic/glycolic acid)
- Mineral/physical (a.k.a. zinc oxide-based or titanium dioxide) sun protection
- Skin-reparative peptides
- Hyaluronic acid and skin-plumping ceramides
- Retinol (unless pregnant or breastfeeding)
- Potentially some retinoids (much stronger than retinol), which come in various forms/strengths/levels of irritancy, and are the holy grail of anti-ageing

**IN YOUR 50s AND BEYOND**

- Use a creamy cleanser morning and night
- Use antioxidants each morning to protect the skin
- Maintain healthy cell renewal with regular AHA exfoliation
- Wear SPF 30 each day (in addition to, or in place of, moisturiser) on face/neck/chest/hands
- Use retinol-based anti-ageing serums to target pigmentation, sag, wrinkles and loss of firmness
- Consider professional treatments and services (e.g.: peels, laser, fillers, botox, skin-tightening)
- Counteract dryness caused by decreased oestrogen levels with a peptide-rich night cream (down to the boobs), replenishing face oils and hydrating masks
- Use a nourishing eye cream
- Moisturise your whole body each day after you shower

**Things to look for:**

- Antioxidants (coenzyme Q10, green tea, idebenone, resveratrol, vitamins E and C)
- AHA chemical exfoliators (lactic/glycolic acid)
- Mineral/physical (a.k.a. zinc oxide-based or titanium dioxide) sun protection
- Peptides and ceramides
- Retinol or Retin-A
- Hyaluronic acid and glycerine for nourishment

# A SUGGESTED GENERIC DAILY SKIN CARE ROUTINE IF YOU'RE IN YOUR <u>TEENS.</u>

## Remember:

Not all sun protection is the same, and the type you use will influence your morning routine. If you're using a moisturiser with chemical sunscreen, apply it onto clean skin, then follow with makeup. If you're using a physical sunscreen (zinc oxide or titanium dioxide based), apply serums/oils first, then your daily moisturiser with sun protection, primer, then makeup. Basically stuff that needs to be absorbed (treatment serums and chemical sunscreens) must go on skin first, and barriers (like face cream, physical block sunscreens and makeup) should be applied last. **I have done the following recommendations based on physical sunscreen.**

### AM

- Cleanse
- Non-oily daily moisturiser with sunscreen

### PM

- Cleanse and remove makeup
- Non-oily/non-comedogenic moisturiser with antioxidants

### Some products to try:

- Teen Aspect Cleanser
- ASAP Clear Complexion Gel
- Clinique Anti-Blemish Solutions Oil-Control Cleansing Mask
- Treatments such as blue-light Omnilux, microdermabrasion and peels are good options for acne

# A SUGGESTED GENERIC DAILY SKIN CARE ROUTINE IF YOU'RE IN YOUR 20s.

**AM**

- Cleanse
- Antioxidants
- Moisturiser with physical SPF 30 sun protection

**PM**

- Cleanse/remove makeup
- Exfoliate with AHAs 2–3 times a week
- Hydrating/treatment face oil or serum
- Antioxidant-rich moisturiser (down to the boobs)

**Some products to try:**

- ASAP Gentle Cleansing Gel
- Go-To Very Useful Face Cream
- Invisible Zinc Tinted Daywear SPF 30
- Biologique Recherche Lotion P50V or PCA Skin BPO 5% Cleanser for breakouts

# A SUGGESTED GENERIC DAILY SKIN CARE ROUTINE IF YOU'RE IN YOUR 30s.

**AM**

- Cleanse
- Antioxidants plus relevant treatment serums
- Moisturiser with physical SPF 30 sun protection

**PM**

- Cleanse/remove makeup
- Exfoliate with AHAs 2–3 times a week
- Serums/active treatment products
- Face oil
- Antioxidant-rich moisturiser (down to the boobs)
- Optional: eye cream

**Some products to try:**

- Gernétic Synchro
- Go-To Exfoliating Swipeys
- Aspect Exfol L
- PCA Skin C-Quench Antioxidant Serum

# A SUGGESTED GENERIC DAILY SKIN CARE ROUTINE IF YOU'RE IN YOUR 40s.

**AM**

- Cleanse

- Antioxidants plus relevant treatment serums

- Moisturiser with physical SPF 30 sun protection

**PM**

- Cleanse/remove makeup

- Exfoliate with AHAs at least 3 times a week

- Serums/active treatment products (with retinol, probably)

- Face oil

- Antioxidant-rich moisturiser (down to the boobs)

- Optional: eye cream

**Some products to try:**

- Olay Regenerist Micro-Sculpting Serum

- SkinMedica Retinol Complex 0.5

- Clinique Take The Day Off Cleansing Milk

- Cosmedix Opti Crystal Chirally Correct Eye Serum

# A SUGGESTED GENERIC DAILY SKIN CARE ROUTINE IF YOU'RE IN YOUR 50s AND BEYOND.

**AM**

- Gentle cleanse

- Antioxidants plus relevant treatment serums

- Moisturiser with hyaluronic acid and peptides

- Physical SPF 30 sun protection

**PM**

- Cleanse/remove makeup

- Exfoliate with AHAs at least 3 times a week

- Treatment product with retinol/retinoids

- Face oil

- Nourishing antioxidant-rich moisturiser (down to the boobs)

- Optional: eye cream

PLUG!

**Some products to try:**

- Sodashi Nourishing Repair Treatment

- Estee Lauder Perfectionist [CP+R] Wrinkle Lifting/Firming Serum

- Jan Marini Age Intervention Retinol Plus

- Go-To Face Hero

# HOW TO CHOOSE A MOISTURISER.

Your daily moisturiser has a fairly simple set of objectives: seal in moisture, and hydrate, protect and soothe the skin. In my opinion, most of the heavy lifting should be done by serums or face oils, and a moisturiser should do just that – moisturise. Depending on what kind of skin you have, and what level of moisture is needed, of course. Sounds confusing! Don't worry, it is confusing, so you heard right. Here's some assistance.

## WORK OUT YOUR SKIN TYPE

Find a good facialist or beauty therapist you trust to develop a relationship with (a good skin therapist should become as trustworthy and dependable as your hairdresser), or see page 14.

## CONSIDER THE RIGHT TEXTURE FOR YOUR SKIN TYPE

Oily skins might prefer a lightweight (water-based) lotion or gel, dry skin a thicker cream, ointment or balm-type texture, and normal skins a regular cream.

## BUY A MOISTURISER THAT CATERS TO YOUR SKIN TYPE, BUT ALSO TO WHAT YOUR SKIN NEEDS

Needs are individual, and based on what your skin is lacking or what you would like to improve. Here is a large blue squid. No, wait. Here are some examples:

**Sun protection?** Every one of you, no matter what age or skin type, must be wearing broad-spectrum sun protection, preferably SPF 30, each day. The easiest way to get around the confusion regarding layering is to find a great moisturiser and sunscreen in one, and read page 31.

**Wrinkles?** Buy a moisturiser targeted to mature or ageing skin, which will generally be extra nourishing. Layer it on top of some AHAs or retinol/retinoids, or buy one that includes these ingredients.

**Sensitive?** The less ingredients, the better. Try organic or irritant-free. Face creams lacking the usual 'nasties' (synthetic ingredients and irritants) will be your best bet.

**All skins, but especially young?**
I believe every moisturiser should contain antioxidants (such as vitamins A and E, green tea, resveratrol, idebenone) to protect the skin, and neutralise the free radicals that lead to premature ageing.

**Dry?** Creamier textures with ingredients like hyaluronic acid will lock in moisture. (Applying hydrating serums and/or face oils before your face cream at night will *really* help, as they strengthen the lipid barrier.)

**Acne?** Specific acne-targeted skin care is key (try brands like ASAP and Alpha-H), but definitely go for something with AHAs (like lactic or glycolic acid) and BHAs (salicylic acid).

### HOW TO KNOW IF IT'S DOING ITS JOB
Your skin will feel and look 'good'. Healthy, rejuvenated, happy. Not tight, dry, greasy, or like you're tired. THIS WILL NOT HAPPEN IMMEDIATELY. Most skin care takes a few *weeks*, not days, for results to come through. (I never rave about a cream or serum until I have used

it for 3–4 weeks.) Especially if you're looking for improvement on acne, fine lines or pigmentation. Of course, if you're experiencing any irritation or tightness, then stop and switch.

### DO YOU NEED A SEPARATE NIGHT CREAM?
If your day cream is a moisturiser with SPF, then yes, because you don't need sun protection at night. I recommend buying an antioxidant-filled facial moisturiser without sunscreen you can use on your face and neck morning or night, under makeup, sunscreen, during a long flight, after sun – whenever. (I created my own, Go-To Very Useful Face Cream, for this very reason.) (Sorry! Sorry. I couldn't help myself.)

# A REAL QUICK BEAUTY ROUTINE FOR LADIES WITH LESS THAN 10 MINUTES.

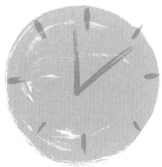

For women who have a 'severe lack of time' or are 'more honest' and admit they may be 'slightly lazy', here is a simple daily beauty routine you can learn and do with flair and ease. First, gently cleanse your face to get rid of any residue oil and prep the skin. Next, apply a moisturiser with SPF 30 (see page 31) every single day, right down to the boobs.

1 Use a BB or CC cream all over the face and apply a little loose powder on top to set it so it lasts. If you prefer more coverage, apply a liquid foundation. (Liquid and cream products are generally faster and easier to apply than powders.) But *do* use some base – even if it is just a tint: it does wonders for making your face look alive and even-toned. Apply concealer under the eyes and on the eyelids to brighten, and conceal any blemishes/veins.

2 The fastest makeup route to looking 'done', in my opinion, is using some colour and simple items that give big results, so that you look like you expended more effort than you did. (If you have oily skin, you will probably prefer to use powders over creams.)

**Here's the most basic makeup routine I can come up with, and it looks great! It *does*! It really does:**

• Mascara. (More is better if you're wearing little else on the face.) Curl your lashes first.

• Blush on the apples of the cheeks.

• Lipstick or gloss.

**If you want to add a little more:**

• Wash of taupe cream eye shadow over the eyelid

• Brown or black eyeliner along the upper lash line

• Bronzer

**3** Add perfume, pull your hair back loosely into a low bun and add some spangly ear candy. I buy earrings from Topshop, ASOS or Zara and they always make me look like I've spent more time on my outfit than I have.

**4** Check the time. It should be around 5–7 minutes after you started this routine. Which, you will note, is less than 10 minutes. Which, you will also note, means A) my heading wasn't a lie, and B) you walloped it. Well done!

# A SIMPLE AND ENJOYABLE TEST TO DETERMINE YOUR SKIN TYPE.

Obviously you already know All This Stuff, but sometimes reminders are useful.

To determine your skin type, softly wipe a piece of white paper over your face in the morning, as soon as you wake up.

*Bonus trick!*

*You know those toilet seat covers in public toilets? They make for terrific blotting paper. Tear some off and dab away.*

## IF THE PAPER HAS NO OIL, YOU PROBABLY HAVE NORMAL/COMBINATION SKIN

Your skin is likely to be in good shape – supple and plump, medium pores, a smooth texture, good circulation, healthy colour. Depending on whether you veer more towards the oily or dry spectrum, by 5pm you might have an oily T-zone, or your fine lines will be more pronounced, respectively.

**Not so good news:** I'll be honest, it's pretty rosy for you. (Lucky!)

**Good news:** You have the least problematic skin type. (Bragger.)

## IF THE PAPER COMES AWAY WITH OIL ON IT, YOU PROBABLY HAVE OILY SKIN

Your skin might have a shiny sheen, with the pores being visible and often large, and the T-zone constantly oily. You are prone to breakouts and blackheads, and your skin might appear thick and congested.

**Not so good news:** Breakouts and acne are common, and you'll constantly be blotting away shine.

**Good news:** Oily skin has *far* fewer wrinkles and looks younger for longer.

**IF THE PAPER COMES AWAY WITH NOTHING ON IT, BUT YOUR SKIN FEELS TIGHT AND DRY AFTERWARDS, YOU PROBABLY HAVE DRY SKIN**

Your skin might feel tight and dry (and possibly flaky and rough), with no oily zones. Fine lines and wrinkles are probably visible and there is likely to be an overall dullness caused by lack of moisture.

**Not so good news:** Dry skin is more prone to visible signs of ageing.

**Good news:** You get far fewer breakouts and you can counter dryness with gentle, hydrating, nourishing skin care. (See page 16 to make sure your skin *is* actually dry, not just dehydrated.)

**IF THE PAPER COMES AWAY FEELING BAD ABOUT MAKING YOUR SKIN CRY, YOU PROBABLY HAVE SENSITIVE SKIN**

Your skin is likely to be very reactive to environmental factors like temperature, wind, sun, and many skin care and cosmetic ingredients. You may be prone to rashes and inflammation, redness around the nose, cheeks, chin and neck, and thinness of skin.

**Not so good news:** Specialised skin care (very gentle) and makeup (mineral, for instance) is best for you.

**Good news:** A lot of brands now offer product lines with fewer or no irritants.

# IS YOUR SKIN TYPE DRY... OR IS YOUR SKIN JUST THIRSTY?

If you're anything like me (6ft, beard, lanky, loud whistler), your skin goes all rubbish and flaky and dry when you hit cold weather. So you start using thicker products, or ones that say 'dry skin'. But that's where you'd be going wrong. Y'see, it could be that your skin is not really 'dry'; *it's just thirsty*. Dehydrated. Here's the difference between the two:

**DRY SKIN**

If you don't often get breakouts and have never had to worry about oil or shine, you most likely have (normal to) dry skin. Dry skin is genetic, it's a skin type, like combination or oily. Cater to this with skin care that is oil-rich because dry skin doesn't produce enough oil (whereas dehydrated skin is lacking in moisture).

**DEHYDRATED**

If your skin is itchy, tight, flaky, dry and, uh, wrinklier than usual, it's probably just dehydrated. You might get a breakout, or have shine. A common misconception is that oily skin can't be dehydrated. Ha! Haha, I say to that! Lie! You can DEFINITELY have oily skin that is dehydrated. After all, dehydration is caused by external factors (wind, cold, heaters, air-conditioning, over-scrubbing/toning or exfoliation), not by a lack of oil, as with dry skin. It's water your skin wants, water, water, water. (Inside and out.)

**The best thing to do for DRY skin:** Switch to a face cream and cleanser that is designed especially to nourish dry skin (look for ingredients like shea butter, ceramides and jojoba oil). An easier option is probably just to apply some replenishing face oil before your moisturiser each night. Changing to cleansing oil instead of your usual cleanser can also help, as can using a hydrating face mask in place of your night cream 2–3 times a week.

**A simple way to assist DEHYDRATED skin:** Drink lots of water, and add a hydrating serum into your skin care routine. (Look for humectant ingredients like hyaluronic acid, phospholipids and glycerine.) Switch to a milk or gel cleanser, as they're more hydrating (and far less stripping) than foaming or scrub varieties, which I reckon should be avoided anyway.

**Whatever you do:** Do not sit next to the heater like I do. Stupid.

*Bonus trick!*

*Never leave your skin bare for more than a minute or so after cleansing, as it will start to dry out. Immediately apply your first product, be that toner or face mist, serum or face oil, or, if you're ignoring a lot of the great advice in this book, just skip straight to your moisturiser.*

# WHEN YOU'RE OVER 30, HOW YOU WASH YOUR FACE MATTERS.

Still using a foaming or scrubby cleanser? *Oh*. What a pity.

Once you hit 30, you really need to kick that habit. Your skin can't take that kind of abrasiveness – it doesn't bounce back like it used to, and it needs more hydration and TLC.

Between 30–35, the collagen and elastin and all the other good stuff in your skin cells that makes your skin bouncy and youthful and firm and plump and adorable start to slack off in a way that is not dissimilar to uni students faced with a lecture longer than four minutes.

So take a gentler approach. You should never have been tugging and pulling at your skin when you apply makeup, but you especially shouldn't be now. And when it comes to skin care, things soften up a little. Especially with cleansers and exfoliation.

Ditch astringent foaming cleansers for mousse, cream, oil or gel cleansers.

And I recommend stopping physical exfoliation ('face scrubs') altogether, which only reach the top superficial layer of skin, not the deep-seated grime lurking below. Plus they can tear and damage the skin. (Plus, the microbeads they use clog waterways and end up in the ocean, which is shit.) Instead, move over to chemical exfoliators (AHA/BHAs), which are far less aggressive, more effective and *way* more thorough.

**Some cleansers that fit this bill:** Bioderma Sensibio Lait or H2O Solution Micellaire Cleanser; Gernétic Glyco; Clarins Cleansing Milk; Mario Badescu Glycolic Foaming Cleanser.

**And a few exfoliators:** Dermalogica Daily Resurfacer; Go-To Exfoliating Swipeys; Alpha-H Liquid Gold; Olay Regenerist Night Resurfacing Elixir.

PLUG!

# THE BEST CLEANSER YOU'VE NEVER USED.

If you are using an average cleanser at the end of a day in which you have applied things like primers and long-lasting makeup and mineral makeup and sunscreen, you are only doing half the job, and are almost definitely not getting rid of all of the stuff you applied.

Using a cleansing oil (before your cleanser) means all of your makeup is gone (it basically melts it away) so you won't be risking a build-up of grime, which leads to skin that is very unglowing.

Because oil attracts oil, cleansing oils are terrific even if you have oily or blemished skin because they draw out the excess oil and impurities, but don't strip the skin. Any skin type can use cleansing oils. True story.

## HOW TO USE CLEANSING OIL

Your face and hands must both be dry. Spread a few drops of the oil onto your hands and massage over your makeup-covered mug. Wet your hands and massage your face again – the emulsifiers in the facial oil will become milky and you can easily rinse it off. Now you may use your regular cleanser. (If you need it – for some, the oil is all that's needed.)

**Products:** Dermalogica PreCleanse, shu uemura High Performance Balancing Cleansing Oil.

*Bonus trick!*

*Most cleansing oils can be used over the eyes and lashes, but tread softly, as while oil in the eyes isn't painful, it is very, very annoying.*

# ARE WE MEANT TO EXFOLIATE, OR ARE WE NOT?

For years exfoliation (in all its forms) has been viewed as one of the Kings of Skin Care: it clears away dead skin cells, allows all those creams and serums to penetrate the skin properly, and gives you a fresh, glowing face.

But know this: When you use *strong* chemical exfoliants, micro-dermabrasion or peels on your skin, you are removing dead skin cells, yes, but you are also inducing a wound-response system within your skin cells in order to be given a batch of fresh new skin cells. Why do you think you get such gorgeous, fresh skin after these treatments? It's because you have injured (via chemicals, or acids, or physical removal) the top layer of skin cells on your face, and they shit

themselves and quickly start dividing to create fresh new skin cells, because the layer that was doing the job is now in trauma.

Unsurprisingly, we're now realising that too much cell renewal will end up being detrimental to skin health and appearance. Skin becomes thin, worn out and taut, because your skin cells are exhausted. Poor little guys.

So let's all slow it down a little. Let's stop peeling off layers of skin and forcing new ones to come through. Let's still exfoliate gently a couple of times a week, (chemical being my recommendation) because it is beneficial, but overall, let's go easy, man.

### IF YOU'RE UNDER 35

2–3 gentle exfoliations a week is fine. This will gently slough off the (unnessary) top layer of dead skin cells and let your skin care penetrate and do its thing.

I prefer to use a *chemical exfoliant* (clarifying lotions, cleansers or masks with salicylic or glycolic acid) over a physical exfoliant (exfoliating beads/ the traditional 'face scrub') but if you prefer the feeling of a scrub, please ensure the product you use has very gentle, non-plastic, spherical, non-skin-tearing exfoliating granules, and that you massage it in *super gently*.

### OVER 35?

Up it. Do some more. Maybe use an exfoliating cleanser in the shower 3–4 times a week and do a monthly DIY or in-salon micro-dermabrasion or peel. (Try La Prairie's Cellular 3-Minute Peel or Philosophy's The Oxygen Peel.) This is allowed because once you hit around 35, your collagen production starts to decrease and the rate at which your skin cells reproduce slows down, so they need a bit more assistance.

But even then, the gentler, the better. You do NOT want to over peel, over dermabrasion, over exfoliate, over AHA, and end up with crepey, too-thin skin. Cos it happens. You know it does. We've all seen those faces. They're scary.

# YOUR CHEEKS AREN'T CLOGGED. SO WHY EXFOLIATE THEM?

When you apply exfoliant to your face, where is the first place you start massaging it in? Your cheeks! Your lovely, plump, usually blemish- and wrinkle-free cheeks!

Which is silly, because they are the last place your face needs to have dead skin removed. After all, when was the last time someone noticed you have clogged-up cheeks. Feel free to chuckle at this point, because obviously such an idea is just preposterous.

Most of us really only need to be exfoliating on the T-zone, so next time you place that stuff onto your face, don't go for the cheeks, start on your forehead or nose or even your chin, first, and do a light sweep of the cheeks to finish.

# YOUR FACE IS LIKE A SPONGE.

You know how you have to wet a sponge before you can use it, so it will absorb your Cleaning Agent of Choice, because if you try to clean with it when it hasn't been pre-wet, nothing absorbs, and you're just there, wiping a bench futilely, getting none of that spaghetti sauce off?

Well, your face is the same: you need to prep the face in order for the skin to be able to properly receive the next product that goes on – be that your serum or your moisturiser. This prep also serves to thoroughly clear away any debris on your mug, debris that leads to a clogged and dull complexion.

In the old days, when Cookie Monster didn't give two burps about cookies being a 'sometimes food', all we had for this was toner, but now we have a whole plethora of products that beautifully hydrate and prepare the skin for taking in skin care goodness, like facial mists, essences and clarifying lotions.

**If your skin is low on moisture:** Use a specifically targeted hydration product and apply onto dry, clean skin before your regular skin routine. Try SK-II's Facial Treatment Essence, or shu uemura's Depsea Water Facial Mist – both are terrifically hydrating, protecting and energising.

**If you want to soothe your skin:** Try a calming, organic mist, perfect for skin suffering from redness or irritation, or just anyone really. Sodashi Calming Rose Face Mist smells delightful and really aids absorption. Great to mist over makeup to set it, too.

**If your skin is dull or congested:** You need something clarifying and gently exfoliating – usually with AHAs – which will gently remove dead skin cells and *thoroughly* clean skin. Following with sunscreen is CRITICAL. Try: Clinque's Anti-Blemish Solutions Clarifying Lotion or Neutrogena's Alcohol-Free Toner.

**Note this:** All of the above count as prep, and so go on before sunscreen.

# OWN SOME CLOTH MASKS ALREADY.

A lot of women say to me, 'Zoë, how is it that you've managed to spill food down your top and it's only 8.15am?' To which I reply, 'I shall *never* reveal my secrets.'

Another thing a lot of women say to me is, 'Zoë, I don't care for salons or facials. Also, they're expensive. And I'm not going to spend an hour at home faffing about in the bathroom doing a home facial. So just tell me how to cheat a burst of good skin already. And make it fast.'

I like these women. They're honest and they're straightforward, and I respect that. So here's what I recommend: Cloth masks.

For those yet to discover them, cloth masks are one-use facial masks actually not made of cloth, but of a thick papery substance. You pop them on your mug for 10 minutes, then chuck them in the bin. So efficient!

They are tailored to specific needs (e.g. brightening, hydrating, anti-ageing)

and have a high concentration of skin-loving ingredients and antioxidants and hydration boosters and skin plumpers, which is what makes them so ideal for a quick, visible skin lift.

They're wonderful pre and post flight, after time in the sun, a hangover or no sleep, before applying makeup for a special occasion, if you know you're going to have your photo taken a lot, or if you're pretty sure you're going to run into your ex-boyfriend and want to look magnificent.

*Bonus trick!*
Exfoliate the face before using your mask for best results. Moisturise afterwards.

*Bonus trick again!*
The day after using a cloth mask, squeeze out any remaining liquid in the sachet and apply as a serum.

# CAPILLARY PREVENTION TECHNIQUE #228.

Never, never, never, ever-ever-ever-ever EVER do that thing in the shower where you turn your face up to the stream and let the water pound it.

WHY NOT? you demand in that tone you know I hate. I LIKE DOING THAT VERY, VERY MUCH.

**Here's why, yelly:** The water droplets come down with such pressure that you can burst teeny blood vessels and end up with (visible, broken) capillaries on your face. Some people even have *a red region on their face in a faint circle*, which is reflective of the way the showerhead sprays the water down. True. Story. Same applies for your delicate, thin chest area. Obviously, really hot water plus pressure on skin is even worse, so keep shower water tepid, not scorchy.

**Much better:** Face straight ahead or turn your back onto the stream, and only ever splash water from your hands up onto your face. (And make sure it's not too hot.)

*Bonus trick!*

*Relieve facey puffiness real quick by wrapping a few ice cubes in a washcloth and sliding it over your face and eyes for a minute or two. Then, press a warm washcloth onto your whole face for 15 seconds.*

*Bonus trick!*

*When choosing a facial, try to choose one that has heat or a compress involved. The heat or compression beautifully infuses all the products into your skin and the results are better and last longer. Also: feels nice.*

# WHY AREN'T YOU USING A SERUM?

You cleanse.
You protect from the sun.
You moisturise.
But do you *TREAT*?

A treatment product is the most crucial element of a skin care routine, because it targets a very specific concern in a way the stuff above cannot. A 'concern' being the main thing you'd like to improve in your complexion. Be that acne, wrinkles, firmness, pigmentation, dehydrated skin; whatever.

Serums are basically the equivalent of a shot of tequila to your moisturiser's glass of wine: they're concentrated, they're more powerful and they're more effective.

You can begin using a serum in your early twenties (or even earlier if you have problem skin) but they become increasingly important as you age, because, uh, your skin needs more help. You apply them once or twice a day (at night, certainly) directly after cleansing (or toner), and before face oils or creams. Simple.

They're usually more expensive because they use higher doses of actives and are more concentrated. *This is okay.* You can afford to spend less on the rest of your skin care if you have a shit-hot serum, because they are the surest and fastest way to see a noticeable improvement in your skin. Like trolls guarding bridges, they are very good at doing one thing well.

If you have multiple concerns? It's like choosing your shampoo and conditioner when your hair is coloured, dry AND frizzy: go for the concern that is most pressing and, when treated, will make the biggest difference to the look and feel of your skin. Or, choose one of the snazzy do-it-all serums.

*A note on face oils / serums:*

*Face oils are often referred to as serums, but this is incorrect. That said, face oils do offer some of the same benefits, and can be a fantastic substitute if your concerns aren't too specific.*

### YO HO HO AND A BOTTLE OF SERUM

**Value:** Olay Regenerist Micro-Sculpting Serum

**Anti-ageing:** Ultraceuticals Ultra A Skin Perfecting Serum

**Hydrating:** Chanel Hydra Sérum

**Pigmentation:** SkinMedica Lytera Skin Brightening Complex

**Antioxidants:** SkinCeuticals Phloretin CF Gel

**Do-it-all:** Estée Lauder's Advanced Night Repair

**Acne:** Mario Badescu Anti-Acne Serum

**Fictional:** Slick Jim's 100% Genuine Magic Potion

# OUI! YOU CAN LAYER YOUR SERUMS, MADEMOISELLE!

Serums are treatment products; choose them based on your biggest skin concerns. But because the skin gods can be bitchy, sometimes we have many skin concerns at once: dehydration, acne, dryness, sagging and loss of firmness, big pores, redness, hyperpigmentation, and too much icing sugar around the mouth from excess doughnut eating.

Yeees, there *are* do-it-all serums, which are fine for skin that isn't yelling for attention, and yes, face oil *can* act as your 'serum'. But if you have specific issues, go for specific serums, and don't be afraid to layer them, working from thinnest and most active, to thickest.

As an example, here's what I do each morning as a brave woman waging war against pigmentation and dehydration:

1 Cleanse.

2 Apply a pigment blocker, which helps to stop pigmentation from forming in the first place. (I like Aspect Pigment Punch.)

3 Apply an antioxidant serum or oil to protect my skin from free radical damage ('premature ageing'). I like Skinceuticals Phloretin CF and my very own Go-To Face Hero because I am part genius/all bias.

4 Apply a zinc-based physical sunscreen. Physical sunscreens go after serums, remember. Chemical sunscreens, by comparison, go **first** and onto clean skin – making it hard for serums to penetrate, and another great reason to make the switch to a physical.

5 Apply CC cream for coverage.

This routine means I am protected against UV damage and pigmentation, and thoroughly hydrated. Others might use something for controlling congestion and oily pores,  followed by an antioxidant serum, or even a highly active vitamin C serum coupled with a hydrating one for a day where bright, glowing, plump skin is needed more than treatment solutions.

*Some serum dot points:*

- *Layering two serums is fine; three is probably the limit.*

- *Not all serums are good for night AND day – save retinol, retinoids and AHAs for p.m.*

- *Make sure your serums aren't fighting each other, or you're not doubling up on ingredients or benefits, or the accumulation of the ingredients doesn't mean you're giving yourself a mini peel each day. In other words, get professional advice before you purchase/ embark!*

- *Serums can't rollerblade very well and will be embarrassed if you ask.*

# THREE WAYS TO USE BB CREAM OR TINTED MOISTURISER:

**Two:**
Mix it with your face cream and blend it down your neck and chest as a kind of tinted body lotion. (Important when you're wearing skimpy straps/low tops and your face is one shade, your chest another.)

**One:**
Merge it with your regular liquid foundation (in a 30 to 70 ratio) to add a little bit more 'blendability' and, depending on the one you're mixing in, radiance.

**Three:**
Mix it in with your primer (50/50) and use all over your face as a kind of moisturising, illuminating base before you apply powder foundation.

# DOES A MOISTURISER OR FOUNDATION WITH SPF PROVIDE ADEQUATE UV PROTECTION?

It depends **on the kind of sun exposure you'll be getting and how much product** you use.

For the sake of simplicity, let's say that the sun exposure we're talking about is for a regular day, or 'incidental', which means you're not going to go outdoors much, save for getting some lunch or walking to and from the train station.

This amount of UV exposure means as long as you apply it according to the correct amount needed for the SPF to work (see page 34), a daily moisturiser with SPF 15 or higher will do the job.

However: Moisturisers with SPF will often not be broad-spectrum (UVA and UVB protective) and because of all the ingredients in the moisturiser, the ability of the SPF to do its job properly can be diluted. Try to buy one that is water-resistant if possible as its UV protection will be more stable, or better yet, a zinc oxide- or titanium dioxide-based physical sunscreen.

Similar story with your BB cream or foundation: yes, it might have SPF, but relying on it as your SOLE source of sun protection is a bit stupid. Mainly because for you to get the SPF protection on the label, you need to use it at a rate of 2 mg per cm$^2$. Which is a fair amount. And also, few foundations have UVA protection or are photostable. The simple way around all this? Use a daily moisturiser with broad-spectrum SPF 30 every day.

*Fun fact!*
*Plain sunscreen is often equally as emollient as a moisturiser with SPF, but we prefer the scent and feel of face cream.*

*Sun fact!*
*It's hot.*

# SUNSCREEN OR MOISTURISER FIRST?

Depends.

Are you using a **chemical** sunscreen?

Chemical sunscreens ('most sunscreens') absorb the sun's rays into your skin, like a sponge, and feature hard to pronounce ingredients like helioplex, oxybenzone and avobenzone. They must be applied to CLEAN skin to be effective (so, directly after you've cleansed), and require 20 minutes absorption to be effective. It's not recommended to apply additional skin care on top of sunscreen, so you're best off using one with a moisturising base as an all-in-one each morning and be done with it.

**Ticks:** Chemical sunscreens are colourless, odorless and sink in to the skin easily.

**Crosses:** They can be irritating to the skin, and cause allergic reactions. More crucially, some chemical sunscreens are not photostable, which means they breakdown after sun exposure, which leads to free radical damage, which leads to skin damage/ageing/ hyperpigmentation. Or in other words: all the stuff you want your sunscreen to *protect* you from, skin cancer obviously notwithstanding. Also, some are thought to be endocrine disruptors (messing with your hormones).

**Good brands to try:** SunSense, Olay, Cancer Council, La Roche-Posay, Clinique.

...Or are you using a **physical/mineral** sunscreen?

These deflect or block the sun's rays from your skin, like a mirror, rather than absorbing them. They are made from zinc oxide or/and titanium dioxide, and are applied *after* your other skin care, as the final step (just before makeup.)

**Ticks:** Zinc oxide and titanium dioxide are both stable and safe, and start protecting the skin as soon as they're applied. Zinc oxide is ideal for those with sensitive skin.

**Crosses:** Titanium dioxide only protects against UVB, not UVA rays (which is why it's generally accompanied by zinc oxide). Also, these minerals can be thick and ghosty on the complexion. To counter this, companies often use micro or nanoparticles, which, despite criticism, have been proven to be safe. (See page 34.)

My pick?

Physical. I use a daily moisturiser with physical (zinc oxide) SPF 30 sun protection (and antioxidants if possible) every single day, forehead to boobs. I demand stable defense against UV damage, especially since I use a lot of AHAs on my skin, which leaves it vulnerable. Also, as someone who battles hyperpigmentation, knowing that there's a chance chemical sunscreens can trigger inflammation and make my hyperpigmentation *worse* has put me off them.

**Good brands to try:** Aspect, Wotnot, Invisible Zinc, Soléo Organics, Jan Marini.

*Remember this:*
UVA = ageing rays
UVB = burning rays

# OTHER SUN CARE POINTERS YOU'D BE JUST GAGGING TO READ BY NOW:

Many sunscreens now combine both chemical and physical ingredients to ensure a truly thorough barrier against the sun; these make sense. Or, you can do it yourself, layering chemical sunscreen in your moisturiser with high quality mineral makeup, for example.

**Regarding reapplication...** Yes, it says to reapply every two hours. But this is if you have been outdoors in direct sun, or sweating or perspiring. Not sitting inside at a desk. (Although windows can let a heckload of UV in, on aeroplanes as well as in offices.) One way to get around this if you have a full face of makeup on that you don't want to re-do is by reapplying a mineral sunscreen powder all over as needed. (Try DermaQuest or Colorescience.)

**Regarding outdoor/beach/exercise needs...** For sport or swimming, chemical sunscreens tend to be the better choice as they last longer in 'wet' conditions. Ideally, layer a chemical underneath a physical. And reapply, obviously.

**Makeup with SPF isn't enough...** Not even that fancy BB cream with SPF 30. You won't use enough and you won't apply it evenly enough. By all means use foundation with SPF, but layer it on top of broad-spectrum sun protection, ay.

**The amount counts!** You need around ¼ teaspoon for your face, same again for your neck, and, if it's going to be exposed, the same again for your chest. This is the amount recommended to make your sunscreen effective *so do it*.

## Regarding nanoparticles...

*To date, the current weight of evidence suggests that titanium dioxide and zinc oxide nanoparticles (commonly used sunscreen active ingredients) do not reach viable skin cells; rather, they remain on the surface of the skin and in the outer layer of the skin that is composed of non-viable cells. A study published in 2014 exposed human immune cells (called macrophages) to zinc oxide nanoparticles to see how they would respond. The study showed that the human immune system effectively absorbed the nanoparticles and broke them down. The study did not look at whether the particles are absorbed through the skin and into the bloodstream. The current available evidence indicates that this does not happen and the particles remain on the surface of the skin.*
From: The Cancer Council, April 2015.

# FIVE

## Shit weather beauty fixes.

We all know the moment you step out into rain and wind all your grooming is going to turn to hell. And balaclavas, while useful, are generally frowned upon.

So why not allow me, the grand priestess of self-important advicery, to offer you a few stealthy techniques to help you look tasty, not pasty?

### 1.

**Only dinguses wear gloss in horrible weather.** Your hair will stick to it and don't tell me that's not up there with excessively beepy microwaves in the annoyance stakes. Go for lipstick, or lip butter, or lip stains and hydrating tints (which will protect lips from the wind) instead.

### 2.

**Use stains and tints.** A cheek tint is perfect in this weather because it won't budge. It will stay put even if the rain belts down on it (where ARE you? Go inside, for the love of legwarmers!) and you can use it on your lips AND cheeks. I love Benefit Posietint (flamingo pink) or Cha Cha Tint (peachy).

### 3.

**Use all your waterproof stuff.** It's not just for summer, you know. Works real good in the wind, rain and snow. Of course, this mainly pertains to the eyes: mascara, liner and shadow. I like MAC Paints smudged on the eyelids, with waterproof liner and waterproof mascara to finish.

### 4.

**Try the Rich Lady In Winter look.** Blow dry, smooth and style your hair as much as you can be arsed. Use mousse to start, and set it all with a humidity-fighting hairspray or lacquer (John Frieda does one). Pull up the collar on your coat, and jam a chic beanie or hat over your nicely done hair. Style cat! *Meow!*

### 5.

**Focus on the lips.** I am partial to matte lipstick with bronzer and lots of lovely black lashes (waterproof, of course) on a backdrop of full, semi-matte coverage (eyelids included) when the weather is turbulent. Red and wine-coloured lips look devilishly good in winter, but then so do pink and orange, to be honest.

# ON THE TOPIC OF EYE CREAMS...

Some people maintain you don't need a separate product for the eye area because any well-formulated, non-irritating face cream or serum will do the job adequately. (So long as it's not applied any higher than the orbital bone.) Others say that since the eye area is a very 'high expression' area (read: wrinkle-prone), and has very few oil glands (unlike the rest of the face), it most definitely needs additional nourishment, and since eye products often utilise ingredients with smaller molecules, which are able to penetrate the delicate eye area, they are not able to be substituted for thick facial moisturisers.

Whichever eye product you do go for, make sure it works hard, is specific to your needs and won't forget your birthday. And definitely use sunscreen each day. And wear sunglasses. And sexy wink *heaps*.

**If you are young and want to help minimise the onset of fine lines and wrinkles:** Good idea! Wear daily moisturiser with SPF every day and at night, a hydrating eye serum with antioxidants. (Like Sukin Antioxidant Eye Serum.)

**If you are noticing dryness, fine lines and wrinkles and wish not to:** Wear sun protection and choose an eye cream with antioxidants and rich moisturisers (ceramides, peptides and hyaluronic acid ideally); this will protect you now, and down the track. I use CosMedix Opti Crystal Chirally Correct Eye Serum and it's fantastic.

*Fun fact!*
*Serums generally have smaller molecules than creams and will sink into the eye area better.*

**If you have darkness under the eyes:**
This is a real bitch because if it's not
caused by lack of sleep, it could be a
genetic gift from your parents. Or it could
be caused by melanin (pigmentation).
Your best bet is to wear sun protection
on the area daily then something melanin-
inhibiting at night (such as Shiseido
White Lucent Anti-Dark Eye Circles
Eye Cream). Another option is to wear
a hydrating, light-reflecting eye cream
(like MD Formulations Moisture Defense
Antioxidant Eye Cream) then work on
the circles cosmetically with a corrector
(see page 134), then a concealer, then an
illuminator (see page 67).

**If you want to avoid pigmentation:**
Definitely wear daily moisturiser with SPF
(physical, ideally), or a dedicated eye
one, like SkinCeuticals Physical Eye UV
Defense.

**If you have puffiness:** To be honest,
you're better off using your existing eye
cream/serum but making it cold, and
spending a few minutes massaging it in
than spending on a de-puffing 'magic
product'. That said, some products will
be more helpful than others: consider
a gel over a cream (something super
emollient can compound puffiness) and
keep it in the fridge. (Pressing an ice-
cold face cloth or teaspoon on the area
for a few minutes also helps.)

**If you have deep-set wrinkles:** Buy
exfoliating/nourishing eye creams with
AHAs and vitamin A (retinol) but BE
ALERT! They can be irritating. Options
include L'Oréal Revitalift or Dermalogica
Age Reversal Eye Complex. And of
course: sunscreen.

**If you have a mixture of these delights
or want to cover all bases:** Get an
all-rounder that works on hydrating,
smoothing and brightening the entire
eye area. One option is Aspect Eyelift.

**If you are a pirate and have a rash
from your eye patch:** Yarr! Ye deserve it,
ye mutinous, scurvy-infested sea dog!

# FADE DARK SPOTS AND BRIGHTEN YOUR COMPLEXION TO LOOK YOUNGER.

Wrinkles and lines aren't the only thing making us look older; uneven skin tone (that is, age spots, pigmentation and sun spots) has a heckload to do with it. And when the human eye sees an even-toned, luminous complexion, we immediately calculate a younger age, and a healthier person.

Think of those older people from parts of the world who see little sun (say, Poland) who have plenty of wrinkles, but because their complexion is flawlessly even, the overall appearance is one of luminosity and health. See? You're starting to get it now, aren't you? (Polish metaphors always do the trick.)

**A RUN-DOWN ON SKIN BRIGHTENING**
Brightening/whitening products are designed to break down the clusters of melanin that cause freckles and pigmentation and brown spots. They'll

also – as a bonus for being nice enough to purchase them – brighten your skin all over, and tease dull, uneven skin so much so that it ups and leaves, taking its ball with it.

Brightening the skin is CRUCIAL if you wish to appear more youthful. Sure, work on those lines too, but there is little point having crease-free skin if it's covered in pigmentation and dark spots, which are caused by things like UV damage, hormones (e.g. the mask of pregnancy women get around the forehead and eyes during pregnancy, or while on the pill) or post-inflammatory pigmentation, which is when you've picked at a pimple and you get a scar.

**Annoying truth:** Dark spots and pigmentation are a P in the A to get rid of. Took you years to get that damage, gon' take you a while to get rid of it.

## YOUR OPTIONS

**Easy and effective:** Wear a pigment-inhibitor serum each morning under your sunscreen. Then follow with a brightening skin care regime at night; most skin care brands offer them these days. Clinique's Even Better Clinical Dark Spot Corrector and John Plunkett's Superfade consistently rate well.

**Very effective, but with a fair whack of effort:** Undergo a series of strong in-salon AHA peels and/or possibly something like DermaFrac to further brighten the skin.

**Requires dedication and money:** A course of IPL (Intense Pulse Laser) or Fraxel is reputed to be a long-term way to remove dark spots and discolouration, but be warned that in some cases the inflammation of the laser can actually make the pigmentation WORSE. Do your research!

## NOT AN OPTION

**Ignoring sun protection:** It is absolutely *essential* for preventing and halting pigmentation. I recommend a zinc oxide/titanium dioxide SPF 30 sunscreen every day. Also, hats and sunglasses and shade.

*Lingo fact!*

*'Brightening' and 'whitening' refer NOT to bleaching your skin, but to fading melanin (the build up of which causes dark spots/pigmentation) and improving the overall tone and luminosity of the complexion.*

# THE BEST WAY TO <u>EXCEPTIONAL</u> LOOKING SKIN.

If your wedding is coming up, or a big event, or you just want skin that is a *rude* shade of health, I highly recommend investing in some LED light therapy, or more accurately, some Omnilux (a brand of LED) sessions. (In Australia, you can find salons with Omnilux via spauniverse. com.au.)

It's terribly effective when combined with a series of traditional facials and peels, and I, for one, bloody swear by it. Shit! (See?)

**WHAT IS LED THERAPY**

A non-invasive form of photorejuvenation that involves lying down under a (VERY) bright lamp for 20 minutes. The skin cells are activated with pulses of low-level, non-thermal light energy, which stimulates collagen production (plump, glowing skin, fine lines diminished), gets the lymphatic system moving (no more puffiness) and rejuvenates and brightens and hydrates the skin.

**IN NON-NERDY SPEAK**

It's like a mobile phone charger for your skin – it boosts your skin cells up so that they're running perfectly again.

**THERE ARE THREE SETTINGS ON THE OMNILUX:**

There's the 'blue' head, which neutralises the bacteria that causes acne and inflammation (an excellent treatment for angry teenage skin), the 'plus' (infra-red) head for deep lines and wrinkles, and the 'revive' (red) head, which treats fine lines and wrinkles, improves elasticity, skin tone and texture. And helps with jetlag. And puts you in a good mood. I LOVE the red happy lamp. It's my pick. *Instant* glow.

**FOR THE BEST EFFECT**

Do a program of 1–2 Omnilux sessions a week, combined with a program of light peels and facials, for at least three weeks. (This will not be cheap – each session under the lamp is around $90.) Complement with good skin care at home and kaPOW, suddenly you're wearing less makeup, glowing wildly and attracting more compliments than a celebrity in a sea of sycophants.

**IMPORTANT NOTE**

There is no down time, no UV rays, lasers, needles, pain, or anything that can possibly burn or injure your skin. The whole experience is just lovely, in fact.

# JUICE UP YOUR LAUGHTER LINES.

As adorable as they are, sometimes we do not wish our laughter lines to be visible. Here's how to lessen their appearance, without botox, fillers or needles of any kind. (Not even knitting ones.)

• Make sure you've had plenty of sleep and water. Hahaha! Oh come on, we all love a laugh; that's how we got those lines in the first place.

• Exfoliate your skin so that any dead skin cells are removed (they make fine lines more pronounced).

• Use a hydrating and regenerative face cream at night.

• Use a serum with hyaluronic acid to plump and hydrate.

• Use a nourishing eye cream, patted in all around the eye.

• Use a silicone-based line-filler on the lines before your makeup, or afterwards, depending on the product.

If you find your laughter lines have become more pronounced as the day goes on (from not drinking enough water, air conditioners or working in the Antarctic), gently warm some face oil between your fingers and press it onto the creased area (even over your makeup). This will instantly freshen the area.

If you are touching up your makeup at your desk before a dinner date, dab some more eye cream on the area before adding creamy concealer.

# A SLINKY, SILKY WAY TO KEEP WRINKLES AWAY.

Do you know how much of a difference it makes to the lines on your face in the morning if you sleep on a silk pillow versus a cotton one? Also, have you ever considered caviar for breakfast and giving up that Mazda for a brand-new Ferrari? I jest. But not about that pillowcase.

Y'see, when you sleep, your skin can be prone to wrinkling and stretching and creasing, and with cotton (and God forbid, synthetics) your skin can snag on the material and when it creases, your skin creases with it, like a sick little wrinkly dance. But when you use a *silk* pillowcase, this won't happen. The soft, slidey texture means no folds and alleviates the strain on the skin. Your face glides all over the pillow like an expensive yacht floating over a sea of French champagne.

What's that? I'm being a snob again? *Giles!* Switch on the anti-snob device, would you? Also, prepare me some foie gras! At once!

For me, the proof is not in the pudding, but it IS in the mirror: no longer are there lines sprawled across my face when I wake up.

# USE CLAY TO MAKE SPOTS GO AWAY!

What's that you clay? Ha ha ha! Great job, Fosters. Take five.

Clay is excellent for drawing out oil and impurities and gently tightening pores.

One way to harness its power is on congested skin. Cleanse and then steam your face (large bowl, boiling water, tea towel over the head) for 10 minutes before using a clay mask (like Aveda Deep Cleansing Herbal Clay Masque). Do it a couple of times a week for best results.

For wicked solo pimples that arise to ruin a lady's day, go for a thick clay paste, and it is here that I must gently yet aggressively push you towards the Ultra Famous and Beauty Editor-Loved Payot Pâte Grise. It's a little pot of clay paste that smells and looks pretty vile, which you dab on the offender (after cleansing and toning with a zit-zapping lotion containing salicylic acid for the best results) before bed. It calms redness and inflammation and elegantly draws out the whitehead, so you can hygienically and cleanly pop it (using a tissue, not your fingers) in the morning. But sometimes it clears the pimple right up with no need for extraction! *What a guy.* Thanks, Payot.

I occasionally use it VERY THINLY during the day, because as well as gently drying out the spot, it kind of acts as a concealer too. But you must be careful doing this, because remember, *it's drawing the pimple out*, so by 2pm you might have a walloping great whitehead on your chin, and no way of cleanly and carefully removing it.

One superproduct that has both the drying lotion AND clay in one is the exceptional Mario Badescu Drying Lotion. God it's good.

# PIMPLE TREATMENT PRODUCTS GO ON <u>BEFORE</u> YOUR MOISTURISER.

Similar to rocket science or peeling a grape, the order of zit-killers and face cream is something you never really learn in life. So learn it now, why don't you?

1 The pimple solution/treatment gear should be applied on clean skin so it can penetrate, and do its job without interference from other products. So, you'd clean your skin and then apply your benzoyl peroxide or salicylic acid topical cream on the pimple. (The angrier, more 'blind' painful spots are better treated with benzoyl peroxide over salicylic acid.)

2 *Now* apply your moisturiser. (The less irritating/less fragranced the better.) Don't be fooled into thinking pimples should remain unmoisturised so they can dry out. That's daft. The pimple solution is already drying the Shirley Temples out of it; to further dry out the spot means you'll get dry, flaky skin, which makes everything look worse and more noticeable.

3 If you need to go out, gently apply a medicated concealer/blemish stick with a concealer brush (so as not to spread bacteria to the concealer). A touch of powder on top will set it real nice, especially if it has a shiny, angry whitehead that keeps shining through.

4 If you don't need to go out, leave it well alone and come back to our Uno game already. We've been waiting for ages, spothead!

*Bonus trick!*

*When you get scars from past pimple picking, trying to fade them with vitamin E-type oils won't work. It's pigmentation! Post-inflammatory inflammation! Different to a scar. Use glycolic acid-based products to brighten the skin instead; treat it as you would any other type of unwanted pigmentation.*

# HOW DO I DEAL WITH HORMONAL BREAKOUTS?

*Disclaimer:*

*There may be a disclaimer coming.*

*Disclaimer:*

*Hormonal breakouts, as their name implies, are caused by hormones. So while I can offer some topical solutions, unfortunately the pill is sometimes the only true fix.*

*If your skin has flared up because you went off the pill, or the breakouts are on the chin and jaw (where hormonal spots hang out), or if it's worse on or before your period, this might be of some help:*

**1** Switch to a salicylic or glycolic acid-based cleanser and have a benzoyl peroxide zit-zapper on hand to spot-treat pimples. (I've spoken of my love for Mario Badescu Pimple Drying Lotion many times. Won't mention agai—. Oh, shit.)

**2** Controlling all that oil can dry out the skin, so make sure your face cream is gentle and nourishing, but not too heavy. A lightweight face oil can also do wonders.

**3** Peels that incorporate AHAs and BHAs will be fantastic for you (brands like ASAP and Alpha-H excel here). Clay-based masks also work very well.

**4** A course of AHA peels (to control oil and dirt) and some blue-light Omnilux lamp sessions (boasting anti-inflammatory and anti-bacterial properties, to keep the sebum from causing too much strife in the pores, and getting infected and carrying on) can be very effective. Not cheap. But effective.

**5** Sometimes, the only way to get your skin and hormones in check is the pill. I can't advise which one you should take because I didn't go to Doctor School, nor can I personally recommend it because even though my PMS is epic, I could set fire to a house of kittens when I'm on the pill. So I avoid it. I take supplements with chaste tree berry (Estro-Sense by MD Nutritionals) and evening primrose oil to calm the wild beast instead.

# LOOK PRETTY EVEN AFTER A 14-HOUR FLIGHT.

It's hard to look human/decent/alive when you get off a lo-o-o-n-g flight, because chances are you are *not* Angelina Jolie and thus do not have access to a private jet, and as such, you have spent the last (insert amount) hours with your head pressed against your right elbow/zizzled on Temazepam/watching shitty movies and crying quietly because we all cry watching movies on planes for some reason.

But now it's 23 minutes till landing, and you want to look a bit fresher than you do currently, which is one fruitly short of a rotten banana.

Quick smart, grab your toiletries baggy and get to the dun! *We don't have much time!*

- Splash your face and dry off.

- Massage in face oil and/or face cream.

- Apply some BB or CC cream for glow.

- Dab some cream blush onto the apples of your cheeks.

- Use creamy concealer under eyes and around the nose.

- Use two eye drops per eye.

- Apply stupidly shiny gloss to attract all attention away from bleary eyes.

- Apply some deodorant, you little stinker.

It LOOKS like a long list, but it takes around 2 minutes, and you don't really even need a mirror. This leaves you 21 minutes to wish you'd brushed your pegs before descent or at the very least bought some chewing gum in Singapore.

## Sunscreen on a plane!
*(Like snakes on a plane, but with fewer snakes and more SPF.)*

*Did you know there is a ton of UV rays coming through aeroplane windows? I was a little bit surprised when I learned this, because the first thing I do on a plane is remove all makeup and pop on a gooey hydrating face mask, but, clearly, I am a moron.*

**Point:** *When flying through the day, wear sunscreen.*

# WHEN YOU ACCIDENTALLY FIND YOURSELF AT A LOVER'S HOUSE AND NEED TO LOOK PRETTY IN THE MORNING.

**Brace yourself for a beauty routine that even prisoners of war would reject:**

• Take your handbag into the bathroom – you'll need your makeup.

• Your first move should always be to find any available facewash/scrub and moisturiser, and use that. Have a poke around; most men have at least some Nivea for Men behind all of those bottles of Brut and Blue Stratos. If they don't have that . . . sneak into the kitchen and use some olive oil on a tissue to clean your makeup-soaked mug. Seriously. Avoid soap at all costs: not only has that thing been lovingly rubbed all over pits and dangly bits, it's so harsh on your skin.

• For moisturiser, you could use more olive oil, or something plain like Sorbolene or Vaseline cream body lotion. Stay several kilometres away from the eye area.

• Use mouthwash or rub toothpaste over your teeth with your fingers, do whatever you can with your hair, put on some blush, mascara and concealer, and get out of there already.

*Bonus accidental sleepover trick!*

*It might feel like a bit of a pre-emptive strike, but if you think there's a chance you might end up at a Certain Person's House after a night out because you two have been foolin' around quite a bit lately, pack some face oil in your handbag. It's small, efficient, gets on well with mobile phones and you can use it as a cleanser (with a wet face cloth), an eye cream, face cream and even massage it on as a quick facial if you're drunk and fear hangover skin. And it won't piss your skin off either – it's anti-irritant and works just as well on oily skin. Brilliant. Obviously my very own face oil, Go-To Face Hero, is the one I recommend, but I can't be trusted, so ignore me.*

PLUG!

# THE PRODUCTS TO KEEP AT THEIR PLACE.

Things are going well, huh? Good for you, you loved-up little lamingtons. Now. Time to ship in some loot. You can't be expected to cart around toiletries every time you stay over.

**Facial wipes:** for lazy/late/liquored-up nights. Aim for ones that cleanse *and* remove makeup.

**Cleanser:** something creamy and simple (the cheaper the product, the more you should avoid foaming, because low-quality cleansers use foaming agents as filler).

**Moisturiser:** a non-SPF, non-night, non-specific face cream.

A travel-sized **dry shampoo:** to fake fresh hair The Next Morning.

**A toothbrush:** for your ears, obviously.

Travel minis of **body lotion**, **deodorant** and **body wash**.

Things like tampons, fragrance and curling irons come in a little later.

Things like your spray tan tent and personal sauna, later still.

# LOVE YOURSELF SICK BEFORE YOU LEAVE THE HOUSE EACH DAY.

What's the point of using all that fancy skin care and doing all that hair styling and makeup if you don't take a few moments to admire your handiwork? Replenishing and protecting your skin then ornamenting it with fun colours is a ritual of self-love, whether you recognise this or not.

Oh, *come on*. It is! It's *much* more than a perfunctory daily routine; it's loving and caring for your skin, and making yourself look great, which in turn makes you feel good.

So. I challenge you to think of your daily beauty ritual as less of a necessity and a P in the A, and more of a little moment for you each day where you actively look after yourself, and create a version of yourself, no matter how simple or glamorous, that makes you happy.

Also, have you ever considered full-size cardboard cut-outs of yourself in your bedroom you can kiss goodnight before bed?

But seriously.

Be proud of your eye shadow skills!

Be impressed by your blow drying!

Be grateful for the products you like and which do good things!

High-five yourself (figuratively or in the mirror, your call) for wearing sunscreen!

Thank yourself for bothering to curl your lashes even though you're not convinced you're doing it right/it makes a difference!

Salute yourself for putting in all of this dingin' effort each day!

**It's worth it**: taking pride in your body and your appearance is a beautiful thing.

Alternatively (or additionally), you could write a love note to yourself on your mirror with a whiteboard marker. I'm partial to: 'Holy shit, you look amazing!'

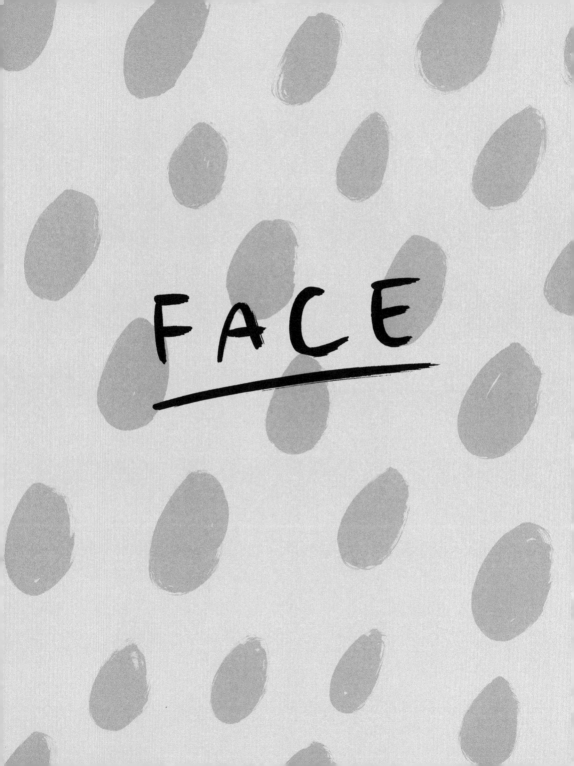

When it comes to makeup, the face itself is incredibly important. Sure, you might have eyes and a mouth, but if you don't have a face to put it all on, well you're really missing out.

Think about it! IT ALL HAPPENS ON THE FACE! The foundation, the concealer, the blush, the bronzer, the illuminator – this is where the magic happens.

The face is the place! THE FACE IS THE PLACE.

# HOW TO TEST FOUNDATION SHADES WITHOUT PROFESSIONAL AID...

...Is by giving them a quiz. They prefer multiple choice but are known to cheat, so be alert and don't leave the room even if you need to go to the wizzer.

Another way to test foundation shades is to select a few you *think* are the right shades and blend them in on the lowest part of your cheek, taking it down to just past your jawline. Now grab your parasol and hitch up your petticoat and step outside. Take out a compact mirror and survey the swiped area in the harsh daylight.

The shade that has disappeared is the right one, and if none has, none is the right one. This means you should go back into the shop and try again, or, if you want my advice (chances are you do, because otherwise you'd be reading *Golfer's Digest*), go to a counter and have a makeup consultant professionally colour match you.

Either way, get it right. You wear this stuff every day, so make sure it's adding to your allure, not subtracting from it by making you look orange or too washed out, or like a teenager who shoplifted the first bottle of foundation she saw and wears it because she wants to feel grown up.

*Bonus trick!*
*If you're faced with two slightly imperfect foundation shades, choose the darker one. Lighter foundations make you look grey, unwell and show up pores.*

# FOUNDATION AS UNDIES, CONCEALER AS CLOTHES.

One question I am asked a lot is, 'Which do you prefer: hot chips, or really hot chips?' Another question I am often asked concerns the order in which a lady should apply her concealer and foundation. Now, some people will tell you it goes concealer, then foundation, but they are wrong, and were probably under the influence when saying such things.

**Apply concealer after your foundation.**
Your foundation's job is to even out the skin tone on your face; so let it. Concealer exists to cover blemishes, or 'fill in' uneven skin tone around the eyes or nose.

Also, since you're just applying final touches, it is far more economical because you'll use a lot less product. Then there's the fact that if you're silly enough to use your concealer first, when you put your foundation on over the top, you'll wipe away all of that concealer anyway.

*Bonus trick!*
*Use concealer around the eye area, not foundation. Concealers have an oil-based texture that suits the eye area, because the skin around the eye has little-to-no oil glands, and this oil prevents the look from becoming cakey, and makes it look smoother.*

# MY TRIED AND TESTED FOUNDATION RECOMMENDATIONS.

When it comes to choosing a foundation, we all have different skin and needs and wants and blah blah blah, but if there's one thing I know, it's my five times table. And also that sometimes, a lady just wants a straight-up recommendation, you know?

**If you have blemished skin:** Make Up For Ever Ultra HD Foundation, bareMinerals Original SPF 15 Foundation.

**If you have a thing for semi-matte, flawless skin:** Chanel Vitalumière Aqua Ultra-Light Skin Perfecting Makeup, Maybelline Fit Me! Dewy+Smooth Foundation.

**If you have rather dry skin:** Hourglass Veil Fluid Makeup SPF 15, Bobbi Brown Moisture Rich Foundation SPF 15.

**If you have a thing for full coverage:** MAC Studio Fix Fluid SPF 15, Clinique Beyond Perfecting Foundation + Concealer.

**If you have sensitive skin:** DermaQuest Liquid Mineral Foundation SPF 30, Colorescience Sunforgettable Mineral Sunscreen Brush SPF 30.

**If you have oily skin:** Laura Mercier Silk Crème Oil Free Photo Edition Foundation, Too Faced Born This Way Foundation.

**If you have skin that is ageing and lined:** Lancôme Teint Visionnaire Skin Correcting Makeup Duo, Covergirl + Olay Simply Ageless Foundation.

**If you wish to have skin that radiates and glows:** NARS Sheer Glow Foundation, Giorgio Armani Luminous Silk Foundation.

**If you have rather red skin:** La Roche-Posay Toleriane Teint Fluid, Clinique Redness Solutions Makeup SPF 15.

**If you want sheer, lightweight coverage:** NARS Pure Radiant Tinted Moisturiser, By Terry Sheer-Expert Perfecting Fluid Foundation.

**If you don't want to spend a lot of cash:** Revlon Nearly Naked Makeup, L'Oréal Nude Magique BB Cream.

**If you have pale and glittering skin:** You might be a vampire.

# WHAT YOU USE TO APPLY YOUR FOUNDATION: IT MAKES A DIFF.

'Always apply your foundation with your fingers!' I used to squawk. 'It warms it up so it melts into the skin and the finish is more natural-looking.'

Look, I concede it's fast and you can get a lovely second-skin look. And some foundations actually *need* the heat of your fingers (many in the NARS camp, for example). But there is something to be said for using a foundation brush*, or a new-gen makeup sponge**, or toast. Sorry, ignore that toast bit. Just a bit peckish.

I use these for foundation because it means:

• I get a (much) longer-lasting effect.

• I get precise application.

• I only apply product where I actually need it.

Unless you have acne, a breakout, substantial pigmentation or redness and need more coverage in more places, all your foundation should be doing is evening out your skin tone. Spend your cash and time on getting your skin in the best condition possible – skin care, facials, exfoliation, sunscreen, peels – so that your foundation need only create a good, uniform canvas for your colour cosmetics, rather than act as a mask.

Oh sure, you can drop $120 on a shithot fancypantsy foundation, but if the skin underneath it is dry, clogged or dull, you will never get the finish you dream of.

**HOW TO DO IT:**

1 After skin/sun care and primer, squirt your foundation onto the side of your wrist above the thumb. Get wild and mix in different tones or types of foundation, or add in luminiser, bronzer or BB cream if you desire.

2 Dab your foundation brush into the mixture and begin 'painting' it on your face. You can layer as needed, but go gently at first and see how accurate and smoothly it applies. Remember: you don't need to take foundation all the way to the jawline, just begin around the nose and move out as required to even out the tone. You *may* only need some on your T-zone and cheeks.

If you're using a sponge, dampen it first, dip it into the foundation, then dab it onto your face. This is especially good for those after a sheer, luminous finish. The 'airbrush' finish will dazzle friends and enemies alike.

3 For creamy under-eye concealer, consider applying with a (clean) fluffy blending eye shadow brush, which will give beautiful coverage under and around the eyes, and mask any redness around the nose.

4 Set the face with a dusting of loose/ translucent powder in the areas that need it (generally just the T-zone) and you're bloody done, you legend. Perfectly applied, and just the right coverage (thickness and spatially).

I hear you muttering that I'm bullying you into adding even *more* shit to your beauty artillery, but I assure you that the quality, appearance and longevity of your makeup is directly proportionate to the effort, time and care you expend on it, and the quality of the tools you use. And honestly, once you've mastered the brushing or sponging, it will take you maybe an extra minute more than if you'd done it with your paws. Even more honestly: do you happen to have any toast I can have?

*\* These are semi-stiff, flat brushes that allow you to paint on foundation. I use a Laura Mercier one. Wash with a gentle shampoo and dry it flat once a week.*

*\*\* Small, tear-shaped sponges with a pointed nib and a spherical bottom, which means you can get into very small areas like under the eye, or do large buffing/sweeping work on the cheeks. Plus, they're cute as heck. Try the beautyblender or similar.*

*\*\*\* Apologies. There is actually no \*\*\* in the copy.*

# AS LOVELY AS A RED, FLUSHED FACE IS...

Let's have a back-up plan in case we decide maybe we're not so keen on it after all, yeah? Here are some tips to reduce and conceal redness of the face, whether it's full-scale rosacea (an inflammatory skin condition characterised by flare-ups of redness on the nose, cheeks, chin and forehead – particularly common in fair-skinned types who blush faster than you can say, 'I love that dress!' and is unfortunately without a cure at this stage) or just prominent blood vessels.
You know, 'redness'.

1 You are, as a redness sufferer, the person who 'sensitive skin' products were created for. The fewer ingredients, the better (organic and authentically natural products are especially good). Cleanse with warm water, never hot, and no rubbing or harsh scratching.

**Try:** Cetaphil Gentle Skin Cleanser, Pevonia Botanica RS2 Gentle Cleanser, Go-To Properly Clean Cleanser.

2 Since redness is inflammation, it's crucial you treat that with anti-inflammatory serums or face oils.

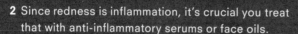

**Try:** Go-To Face Hero, Trilogy Very Gentle Calming Serum.

3 You need face creams that are as hydrating as they are gentle. And you definitely, absolutely need to wear sun protection every single day.

**Try:** Lavera Neutral Face Fluid, Clinique Redness Solutions Daily Relief Cream, SunSense Sensitive SPF 50+.

**4** Correct your skin tone before you apply your makeup
(otherwise you're colour correcting your foundation)
by using a green-tinted corrector on areas that tend
to go red. Not all over. Too Shrek-like. These make a
big difference and take pressure off using too much
foundation to conceal. (If you're VERY pale, perhaps
try peachy/yellow tones instead of green.)

**Try:** L'Oréal Paris Studio Secrets Anti-Redness Primer,
Dermalogica Redness Relief SPF 20.

**5** Use very gentle makeup, preferably a high-quality
mineral, which is not only gentle and loving and
healing for the skin (thanks, zinc oxide) but contains
added sun protection (again, thanks, zinc oxide.
You're terrific. You really are!).

**Try:** Jane Iredale Amazing Base Loose Mineral
Powder, bareMinerals SPF 15 Original Foundation,
ELES Luminous CC Cream 20.

**6** To conceal targeted redness areas, or conceal
flare-ups that occur, touch up with a thick concealer,
foundation stick or powder with a yellow base to
counter the redness.

**Try:** Laura Mercier Secret Camouflage, Shiseido Stick
Foundation Control Color, Glo Minerals Redness
Relief Powder.

# CONCEALER: THE MISUNDERSTOOD PRINCESS OF MAKEUP.

You know that person in your group of friends who is terrific when she's in good form, and a pain in the arse when she's in bad form? In the friendship circle of makeup, this would be concealer. She's magnificent when she's treated well and correctly applied, but is a devilish saboteur when she's not.

Here's how to treat the lady right:

**YES!**
Use a thick, waxier concealer to cover blemishes, sunspots and capillaries.

**Try:** Laura Mercier Secret Camouflage, MAC Studio Finish Concealer.

**NO!**
Don't use that same waxy, thick concealer around the fragile eye area – it is far too dry and won't spread, which means you'll drag and tug at the skin.

**YES!**
Try a do-it-all concealer and see if it works for your needs (dark circles, redness, blemishes, hickeys...)

**Try:** Makeup For Ever Full Cover Concealer, bareMinerals SPF 20 Concealer.

*I nose a real good trick...*

*Next time you apply your makeup, apply concealer (or even under-eye illuminator) around your nose, just on the sides where the nose actually sticks to your face. See? See the difference it makes? Makes your face look lighter, more awake, more even, more flawless and more Absolutely Ravishing because you are evening out shadows and eliminating any redness.*

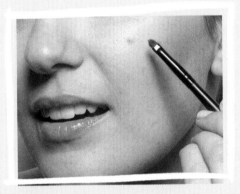

**YES!**

Use a small, synthetic concealer brush to apply precise, small feather strokes over blemishes.

**Try:** BECCA Spot Concealer #32 Brush.

**NO!**

Do not use your fingers, as the oil from your skin will withhold product (and potentially spread infection).

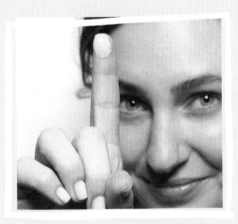

**YES!**

Use a creamy concealer for the under-eye area, and don't be afraid to mix it with some eye cream for a lovely texture. Pat in, don't smear on.

**Try:** Revlon Age Defying Targeted Dark Spot Concealer, ELLIS FAAS Concealer, MAC Select Moisturecover.

**NO!**

Don't nibble on concealer when you're hungry! Eat some grapes instead.

# DON'T PANIC WHEN YOU'RE CONCEALING BREAKOUTS!

If you're over the age of 17, problem skin (the more grown-up term for 'breakouts') becomes centralised, usually on the chin – mainly because our hormones are arseholes. And even though the spots are in one small area, and despite the fact we are Grown-Up Women who should know better, we tend to go silly. After trying to conceal the individual spots, we notice it hasn't worked so well, so we then apply concealer over the entire area to match the spot coverage. All in an attempt to look as though there is NOTHING TO SEE HERE.

**Except we've just made plenty to see here.**

• Next time, just do your regular foundation on the rest of your face and conceal each actual spot (see page 63 on how) with a small-headed nylon concealer brush (Manicare do a great cheap one).

• Upping your foundation coverage, or using too much foundation or powder (usually to match your heavy-handed concealing) is the foible of the panicked and makes for heavy-looking skin, which attracts even more focus. FAIL. You must keep your skin looking luminous and fresh, you confused little cockatoo!

• Avoid powdery textures where possible, use a dewy cream cheek colour and put some focus on the eyes and lips, why don't you.

*Bonus trick!*

*For long-lasting concealer on blemishes, apply loose powder in pale yellow over your concealer with a small shadow brush or mini powder puff. Bobbi Brown has an all-in-one concealer and powder combo that is perfect for such activities.*

*Bonus trick!*

*Make a nasty pimple disappear. With eyeliner. Seriously. Morph any 'focus pimple' (read: large or unsightly) on your otherwise good-skinned face into a beauty mole by covering it in browny-black eyeliner before setting out for the evening. Well done, Copperfield!*

# USE THE RIGHT SHADE OF CONCEALER OR DON'T BOTHER WITH IT.

You will know if you're wearing the Right Shade of Concealer because you won't actually be able to detect it.

This means when you conceal under your eyes, you don't see the whole area become a shade lighter (The Spider Monkey) or small lines of crepey build-up; and when you conceal blemishes, you can't spot them because the concealer is either darker or lighter than the rest of the skin on your face.

Unless you have very pale, fair, pink-toned skin, the best (and by 'best' I mean 'most natural looking') shade of concealer will be yellow based. (This runs true of powder and foundations, too. But not for shoes.) This is because, generally, what we're trying to conceal is purple or blue based – dark circles, post-inflammation pigmentation, capillaries.

Don't forget that the role of concealer in the play that is your daily makeup is to hide imperfections, *not* to colour-correct, lighten the skin or illuminate.

# DETERMINE WHETHER YOU HAVE WARM OR COOL UNDERTONES ALREADY!

It'll help you figure out the most flattering colour palette for your hair colour (see page 174) and makeup and wardrobe, too.

And look, to be honest, I'm tired of waiting for you to figure it out. Got no snacks left. Cold. Tired. Recorded *Real Housewives* and want to go home and watch it.

**IF YOU HAVE COOL UNDERTONES:**

- When you place silver jewellery next to your skin, it's MUCH more flattering than gold

- When you look at the veins in your forearm, they appear more blue than green

- You look better in a pure white t-shirt than a cream one

- You burn but don't really tan

- Your skin could be described as pink, or red based

- You have a bumper sticker that reads: I'M COOL

**Splendid shades for you:** pink, berry, magenta, rose, fuchsia, blue, silver, white, black, blue greens, blue-based reds, blue-purples.

**IF YOU HAVE WARM UNDERTONES:**

- When you place gold jewellery next to your skin, your skin comes to life, as opposed to silver, which is a bit...meh

- When you look at the veins in your forearm, they appear more green than blue (obviously your veins are still blue, but when viewed through skin with a yellow/warm undertone, they look greeny)

- You look better in a cream top than a pure white one

- You can tan easily and when you do, your skin appears golden

- Your skin could be described as peachy, golden or olive

- You look terrific with red or golden, caramel hair

**Splendid shades for you:** peach, coral, yellow, orange, olive green, bronze, brown, orange-based reds, rust, taupe, brick.

# BRIGHTEN UNDER YOUR EYES WITH ILLUMINATOR PENS <u>PROPERLY</u>.

Okay, so you know how you apply your under-eye illuminator/brightener (like YSL Touche Éclat) in a line and then pat it in till it's all gone? Much the same way you do concealer?

There is a much, much better way to brighten the eye area.

**Try this:** Instead of doing a straight line, draw the outline of an upside-down triangle. When you draw your triangle, ensure the base of the triangle is parallel to your lash line, around 1 cm down from your eye, with the pointy bit of the triangle down towards your jaw, on the top of your cheek.

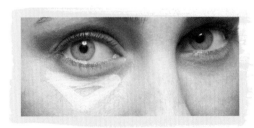

Now, pat it in with a dabbing motion from your middle finger till it's all gone.

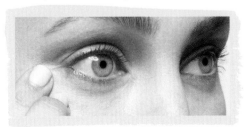

**What you've just done:** Is brighten the *whole* eye area. Y'see, the eye socket is kind of a long oval-circle type shape. So by dabbing in illuminator, you're throwing light on the whole area, and you've blended down far enough that it's totally seamless.

Oh look, it's hard to articulate, but it gives a wonderful effect. Your whole face looks fresher! You'll see.

*Bonus tricks!*

- One thing people get VERY WRONG about illuminators: They are not concealers. *You have to conceal first,* then *use these guys. All they do is brighten.*

- *If you have* serious *dark circles, I recommend using a peachy-yellow corrector first,* then *concealer,* then *illuminator.*

- *Feel free to apply your creamy concealer in an upside-down triangle, too – I do!*

# DO I NEED A PRIMER?
# CUT THE CACKLE!
# TELL ME STRAIGHT!

**IT IS WORTH BUYING AND USING PRIMER IF:**

- Your makeup doesn't last

- Your skin 'eats' makeup

- You need your makeup to last an especially long time (a wedding, a date after work, a day at the races)

- You want some extra luminosity

- You want to 'correct' your skin before applying base

- You don't love using powder

**Know this:** Primer is not moisturiser; it's a preparation agent for a smooth makeup application that will last. Two different things. You'll still be applying your moisturiser (with/and/or sunscreen, of course) before your primer.

**Think of it like this:** Primer acts as a wall between your skin and your makeup. It gives your foundation something to hold on to, rather than your skin. This is why your makeup will last longer – it can't slip into your pores. Primer – depending on which you choose – can also be a masterful problem solver. It can help neutralise redness (green-based), counter sallowness (lilac-tinted), control oil (mattifying), add a healthy flush (pink, luminous) or boost radiance (pearlescent formulas). Your skin care and/or foundation will still do the heavy lifting, but a good primer can certainly help.

Most primers have a silicone base, which kind of sits on top of your skin, and has a velvety, silky feel. This helps your foundation slide on nicely, and creates a delightful, flawless, even canvas for it too. In a seashell, it's a tops product for babes who like even skin tone (colour and texture), and who wear makeup and want it to sit nicely on the skin, for longer.

Not all primers are made equal, though. The one your oily-skinned BFF loves might not work for you, so do some research, try some options and get some advice when buying.

Speaking of some options...

**Mattifying?** I'm a dry cat, not an oily one, but Friends In The Know tell me bareMinerals Prime Time Oil Control primer does an excellent job of keeping makeup in place, and oil and shine in check, like, *all* day.

**Luminosity boosting?** Try Giorgio Armani Light Master Primer, which uses light-reflecting particles to even out and glow-boost even the most tired, drab, uneven skin tones. (No offence, babe, love you miss you mean it xox.)

**Blemish-fighty?** Give COVER FX Mattifying Primer with Anti-Acne Treatment a shot: it contains salicylic acid to fight spots, and helps mattify skin so your makeup stays in place like it dang well should.

**Pore reducey?** A large number of the anti-visible pore army swear by Benefit's the POREfessional, which makes pores less noticeable.

**Hydrating?** Try Napoleon Perdis' Auto Pilot. This was the first primer I ever used and I still use it. It's lightweight and very pleasant on the skin, and will *even* allow you to skip your day cream. (Don't skip sunscreen, though. Stupid.)

**Colour-correcty?** If your skin is on the yellow side, try Smashbox Photo Finish Color Correcting Foundation Primer in Color Balance.

**A bit red?** Try Make Up For Ever Redness Correcting Primer.

**Do-it-all perfection?** If you're at a loss as to which primer to try, you can't really go wrong with Laura Mercier's Foundation Primer Radiance, which has a huge, loyal following of makeup artists and regular bums alike. It blurs and evens out the texture of your skin as well as doing the makeup-stay-put stuff.

*Handy hint:*

*If you wear primer every day (I don't – only when I need my face/makeup to look FULLY SICK and really last) I strenuously recommend:*

*A) A cleansing oil before your regular cleanser for a truly thorough clean (see also page 19).*

*B) Exfoliating 2–3 times a week to thoroughly clean the skin – all that primer will build up, man.*

# AVOID FOUNDATION OR MOISTURISER WITH SUN PROTECTION AT NIGHT.

Sun protection ingredients like zinc oxide and titanium dioxide are opaque, white pigments, which reflect and scatter light rays. This is terrific when we elect not to be ravaged by the sun, but not as great when the sun has racked off, and we wish to have our photo taken, because we think we look delectable, or would simply like to capture and visually document a magnificent evening.

Why? Because when combined with a camera flash, these white pigments make your complexion look white, lifeless and pasty. (Talc can sometimes be the culprit, too.)

*This* is why sometimes you look at photos taken of yourself at parties and square dancing shindigs and cannot understand why your face looks so pale compared to the rest of your body, or despite having a lot of makeup on, and having done lots of clever highlighting, bronzing and contouring work.

**The solution is simple:** Buy a foundation without any sun protection (be mindful that mineral makeup is full of zinc oxide and titanium dioxide) and wear that at night over a simple (non SPF) moisturiser.

# FAKE TAN YOUR FACE; ENJOY WEARING LESS MAKEUP.

Even if you're not self-tanning your body, cos it might be winter and your daily sartorial routine consists of a wool skivvy, some fetching slacks and a pair of gumboots, may I suggest you exfoliate your face and then apply a face-specific self-tanner on a Sunday night (and give it 10 or so minutes to dry) before you apply your night cream?

**WHY I WOULD SAY SUCH A THING:**

When your face is gently tanned (the moisturiser on top dilutes it just so), your eyes appear to be a little brighter, as do your teeth, and for some reason you seem to need less makeup come Monday morning, because your face just looks all healthy and glowy, and to cover it up with a lot of makeup seems criminal.

*Bonus trick!*
*If you have fair hair, run some face cream over eyebrows and the hairline to stop the hair from staining.*

You MUST use a face-specific tanner though, which is why I bothered writing as such in the first paragraph. A tanner for the body is too thick and might very well cause congestion. However, if like me, you have skin that is tough as, you might be able to get away with mixing some body tanner with your face cream and using that instead.

**Try:** Sephora Gradual Self-Tanning Face Water, Clinique Face Tinted Lotion, Santorini Sun Sunless Tanning Face Cream. (Remember, it's your face, so the fewer ingredients the better.)

# HOW TO GLOW WITH THANKS TO LIQUID BRONZERS.

A bronzed sheen, created by a bronzing gel, or a bronze-toned liquid (or cream) illuminator on the cheeks lifts the whole face, and makes you look healthy and glowing, like you've just come off the back off an 8k run and eaten a bowl of organic steamed vegetables. Your eyes look brighter, your teeth so white and TV-advertisement. And! Most brands offer a few shades, from pearly, paler shades right through to dark copper bronzes, so we can all play this game.

You can choose one with a light shimmer through it for a lovely sheen, or go for a more translucent, gel-like, true bronzing gel, which sinks into the skin, leaving a lovely warmth to the face, but no perceptible product. I am more partial to the shimmers at the moment, but last week I wanted non-shimmer. I'm wild like that. Also, some of the shimmers, depending on the opaqueness of the product, are better for night, because walking round with shimmery golden cheeks does not, surprisingly, look that natural and elegant at 11am.

*Fun fact:*

*A little bit of these products goes a L-O-N-G way (some of mine went all the way to Uruguay), so don't baulk at their price. Worth it.*

*Less fun fact:*

*Generally speaking, if you suffer from uneven skin tone (a.k.a. pigmentation) you're probably better off with powder bronzer. Liquid tends to rely on a pretty flawless/even-toned canvas. (Which can be created with base, but you get my gist…)*

**HOW TO APPLY:**

- You can mix some in with your foundation for an all-over glow or apply more like a traditional bronzer (after foundation).

- Use your fingers or a blush brush, which sounds outrageous, but really is such a marvellously simple and effective way to get the product onto your face evenly. Go for a soft, dome-shaped brush if possible. If it's too fluffy and fat, you'll end up with brush strokes and too much all over the cheeks. You need some precision.

- I squirt a blueberry-sized amount on my wrist, and pick some up with my brush, then apply as per powder bronzer (see page 74). Remember: anything with shimmer should sit atop the cheekbones to catch the light.

- Whichever way you choose to apply, look VERY, VERY CAREFULLY in the mirror once you're done to make sure you don't have any streaks. Because being liquid and being quite highly pigmented, this stuff is prone to streaking. (At football games especially.)

- To finish, dab a liquid (like Benefit Posietint) or cream (like Clinique Chubby Stick Cheek Colour Balm) blush on the very fleshiest part of your cheeks, then dust your face with a whisper (shhh) of translucent powder to set the glow without taking any of the freshness away. It won't stay put for very long if you don't. Trust me. I'm a car salesman. I always, always tell the truth.

**OPTIONS:**

**BECCA Shimmering Skin Perfector Liquid** in Topaz – I use this day or night. It's the perfect blend of subtle sheen and bronzer. **Giorgio Armani Maestro Liquid Summer Bronzer** and **Bobbi Brown All Over Bronzing Gel** – excellent for those who want the nice, dewy sheen, without the shimmer. (Making them terrific for day.) They're both a lovely, gel-like texture, and the tiniest amount under and along the cheekbones, temples and forehead instantly wakes up the face. Dark skinned? Try **Revlon Photoready Skinlights Face Illuminator** in Beach Bronze.

# A FUN AND FOOLPROOF WAY TO APPLY BRONZER.

Bronzer is the fastest way for women (and men, for that matter) to look gorgeous and healthy and delicious. However, sadly, most of us apply it incorrectly, because we are yet to read this book and see these pictures.

By brushing your bronzer all over the place, without any thought for the angles of the face or where the face naturally tans, you end up looking overly brown, or orange, or glittery, or muddy. But by doing this simple trick – the 'Double 3' – you look authentically bronzed and subtly contoured.

*Note:*

*There are a few ways to go about bronzer. I have chosen the 'sun-kissed' way, which mimics where the sun would hit, as opposed to the contouring way, which involves Tricky Stuff and is something you should probably investigate on YouTube.*

*Bonus trick!*

*To finish, I sometimes take the TEENIEST amount of bronzer softly down the centre of my forehead, nose and chin, in a side-to-side dusting motion.*

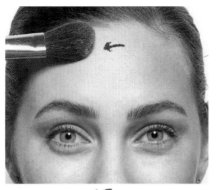

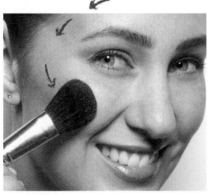

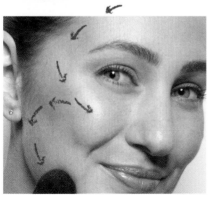

1 Put some bronzer on your fluffy blush brush. Tap off excess. This is important. *Do it.* TAP. Always start off with hardly any product – you can build up the intensity later if you must. That said, **less bronzer is always best.**

2 Place your brush at the top of one side of your forehead, right up near the hairline, and proceed to draw the beginning of a '3' round and down to your cheekbone (acting as the middle of the '3'), going no further than the middle of your eye.

3 Take the brush back to your ear and softly down to make the bottom of the '3' along your jawline, again stopping around the centre of your eye. Blend it in gently so there are no lines.

4 Now, repeat it on the other side of your face. (Obviously on your left side it will be a back-to-front 3.) Go VERY lightly over the top half of the '3' a few times to build colour if you desire, especially around and just above the temples.

5 Marvel at how naturally tanned and flawlessly bronzed your face is.

# HIGHLIGHTERS!
# ILLUMINATORS!
# LUMINISERS!

They have different names and textures (and can often be found sitting alongside a bronzer or blush in a duo for cheeks), but these shimmery, pearlised darlings (different from the creamy pen-style under-eye illuminators discussed on page 67) all do the same thing – accentuate, bring out and enhance a lady's finest facial features. Most notably her cheekbones.

Apply your blush and bronzer before illuminator; it's kind of like the final icing. For powder illuminator, use a small blush brush (too big means too disco face) or a specific highlighting brush, and gently sweep on the product along the very top of your cheekbones (above your blush, not over it) towards your temple.

May I also enthuse the 'Boomerang', where you continue the illuminator up around the eye and under the brow, along the brow bone, in the shape of that most highly sought-after Australian souvenir. If you're using a liquid or cream product, it's a good idea to press the product onto your face with fingers rather than a brush for more accurate application.

*Only use shimmer products if you have good skin.*

Oh pipe down, it's about time there was some common sense applied when women use shimmer products.

If the skin is in fantastic form, GREAT! These products will illuminate and do all the right things. But if the skin is not in fantastic form, shimmer will accentuate lines and blemishes.

**Point:** If you don't have good skin, using concealers to correct flaws (rather than shimmer to draw attention to them) is a much cleverer move.

**Know this:** If you're worried about fine lines under the eyes, skip powder and thick cream illuminators in favour of liquids that sink into the skin instead of sitting on top of it. Also, choose a less shimmery, more 'glowy' formula, to avoid highlighting lines and wrinkles.

**Know this also:** Liquid luminisers can be mixed in with foundation (one-third luminiser to two-thirds foundation) for all-over radiance. Go easy if you have blemished or oily/shiny skin though, as illuminating products accentuate flaws.

**Don't know this:** The exact details of how your parents conceived you.

**Good powders:** Laura Mercier Shimmer Bloc, Bobbi Brown Shimmer Brick, The Body Shop Shimmer Waves.

**Good creams:** NARS The Multiple, Jouer Highlighter.

**Good liquids:** Clinique Up-Lighting Liquid Illuminator, Benefit Girl Meets Pearl.

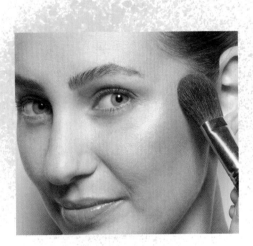

# YOU MUSTN'T BE FRIGHTENED OF POWDER ON YOUR FACE, MY LAMBS!

Loose powder is something I've always eschewed in favour of the radiant, almost-shiny, fresh look I prefer (you know, the one that lasts about four minutes). The thing about loose/translucent powder, for the three of you who don't already know this, is that it's deliberately sheer and lightweight in order to give your makeup lasting power without a powdered look. It's meant to be invisible. Hence the term translucent.

Still, I never used it. Mostly because I was terrified of it settling into my fine lines. But guess what – it WON'T if you apply it right, and use a quality product.

A light dusting of loose powder over dewy foundation and cheek products sets it beautifully all day, and here's a great example of how it can set your painstakingly applied under-eye makeup without making it look cakey.

At this stage you are probably thinking, NO, ZOË! I will NOT! Powder around there will make my fine lines stand out, you naughty little porcupine!

But makeup has come a long way since the days when all powders exacerbated fine lines. The tiny little particles in new loose powders (especially the mineral ones) don't embellish fine lines, they basically fill them in.

You think I'm lying, but I'm not. Hours later, there will still be no fine line creasy business. Suffice to say, if you tire of constantly redoing the under-eye area, this might be a trick for you.

*Bonus tip!*
*Mist your face with a hydrating toner post powder application for an incomparable finish.*

*Bonus tip!*
*Using the word incomparable makes you sound smart.*

**Step one**
Apply corrector
if required, and then
concealer gently
under the eyes.

**Step two**
Follow with an under-eye
illuminator, patting it in up the
inner V onto the eyelid (see page 67),
and all the way under the eye up to the
outer crease, which should always be done
because it can get red and/or shadowy
over there. Pat rather than rub, because
rubbing just rubs away all the product
as well as damaging the delicate
skin around the eye.

**Options:** Nars
Light Reflecting Loose
Setting Powder, Make Up
For Ever Microfinish HD
Powder, Laura Mercier
Translucent Loose
Setting Powder

**Step three**
Take a soft, small
brush or powder puff
with some loose powder
on it, and very gently dab
on some loose powder
over the entire area you
just applied under-eye
illuminator.

# I WAS APPLYING MY POWDER BLUSH WRONG. MAYBE YOU ARE TOO?

Wrong, for the record, means I was trying to do something WAY beyond my capabilities, and for a face I didn't actually own. ('Daryl Hannah in *Splash*.') I was trying to contour and do stuff that girls on YouTube excel at but which mere mortals suck at.

I've since learned an easy, pretty universal technique that you should give a try, or you may die regretting it.

First up, though: **Do not use a walloping great fluffy brush to apply blush**. Terrible idea. Use a small to medium-sized blush brush so you can control the colour and application. (I like a slightly domed one, like Bobbi Brown's Blush Brush.)

I dust my brush over the product (sparingly and always tapping off excess), then smile *pleasantly* (not a big, wide one), and then, using the middle of my eye and the fleshiest part of my cheek as the starting point, I lightly sweep the blush over the apples of my cheeks, and up along the cheekbone towards the top of my ear, stopping a few cm before I get to the hairline. (Sweeping it upwards gives the illusion of lifting and slimming the face. Nice.)

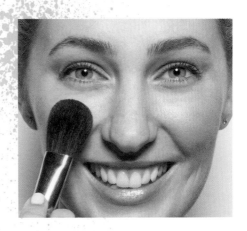

**POWDER BLUSH RECOMMENDATIONS**

**Universally flattering:** Tom Ford Cheek Color in Flush, Shiseido Luminizing Satin Face Color in Petal

**Fairer skin:** Face of Australia Powder Blush in Hello Dolly, NARS Blush in Orgasm

**Olive skin:** Benefit CORALista, YSL Blush Radiance in 03

**Darker skin:** MAC Mineralize Blush in Gleeful, Maybelline NY Fit Me Blush in Deep Rose

*Four extra tips for no extra money:*

1. Never *let your blush sit lower than the bottom of your nose. It makes your face look saggier, sadder and older than it is.*

2. *Whether with BB cream or foundation, it's important to even out your skin tone before applying something with pink/ peach/coral/rose tones to the face, otherwise it can amplify things liked capillaries, scars, under-eye circles, redness and pigmentation. Cute!*

3. *If your blush is too intense, or has made your pigmentation underneath really visible (as can happen), dab on some liquid foundation (with fingers or a sponge) over the offending areas, being careful to blend it properly.*

4. *Keep a product-free blush brush handy to blend out the edges of your blush so that there are no obvious lines, and the finished look is one of a natural, healthy flush, rather than Look Everyone! This Woman Has Applied Blush Today.*

# MAKE CREAM BLUSH LAST LONGER THAN THREE MINUTES.

Cream blush makes the face look fresh, lively and youthful. It's fantastic for those who like a sheer, natural finish, and favour liquid foundation.

Sadly, the very thing that makes it so gorgeous – its texture – means cream blush doesn't stay put very long, preferring instead to steal off and play poker with its loser mates at the pub.

**Here's how to make it last, while retaining a dewy glow:**

Dab your cream blush on to the fleshiest part of your cheeks, and blend out thoroughly.

• Lightly dab on some powder blush in a similar tone – with a medium-sized blush brush – over the cream blush.

• Marvel as your sweet new cheeklets look pink and fun ALL DAY.

• As detailed on page 84, a touch of powder on a cream product is terrific for longevity. In this case, the powder blush on top makes the colour last, but also intensifies the colour while somehow still looking all fresh and flushy and, if we're being crude, just-had-sex-y.

*Bonus trick!*
Use the MAC 188 mini stippling brush to apply cream blush or bronzer, and buff it in gently. (That, or your fingers.)

*Bonus trick!*
Use lipstick as cream blush. Go on, no one's watching. It blends well and looks lovely.

# LAUGH EVERY STONKIN' DAY...BUT DISGUISE THE EVIDENCE.

Is there a way to enjoy blush and bronzer and illuminator without it getting into those crinkles around your eyes? Heck yes. There are *several* ways.

**Fill in any laugh lines with a silicone-based line-filler** before you apply your foundation. It helps create an even base for your makeup and quite literally acts as spac filler. Clarins has one called Instant Smooth Line Correcting Concentrate and L'Oréal has one in their Studio Secrets range, both specifically for laugh lines.

**Pat on, don't rub, concealer under your eyes,** and only apply it where the skin is dark and needs evening out – the inner corner of the eye, under the eyeball and at the very outer corner, leading up to your temple. Everywhere all willy-nilly, and going too low, will just encourage your concealer to settle into lines unnecessarily. (One great solution to this dilemma is Benefit's Fakeup Concealer, which is half concealer, half hydrating magic stick. I love it.)

**Keep blush and luminisers** away from those laugh lines. The less product (especially of the shimmery variety) up there, the better.

**Get rid of your powder blush** (except in the case of gently setting cream blush for longevity, as per the instructions opposite). It settles into fine lines and makes things worse. Instead, buy **cream blush**. Good, well-priced ones come to us via Bloom, Becca, Rimmel, Revlon and Max Factor, and one fancy one that will last and look glorious being pulled from your handbag for (inevitable) touch-ups is Chanel Cream Blush in Chamade.

**If you notice your fine lines getting creasy** (like at 5pm), dab a little face oil onto them, as it'll fill them in and make them glow. (Even over your makeup!)

# THE LIQUID ON LIQUID, POWDER ON POWDER RULE.

Generally speaking: if you use powder foundation, follow through with a powder blush. Liquids and creams, similarly, demand liquids and creams.

**Why:** If you try to put a cream blush, bronzer or illuminator on top of a powder finish, it will grab, and not blend, and you will get cranky, and probably break or throw something or someone.

And if you put a powder blush on your radiant, dewy liquid foundation, it may grab and not spread very well, and a frighteningly similar brand of rage could ensue.

**The exception that makes that rule confusing:** Placing powder gently on top of liquid sets it and makes it last.

**For example:**
• Using a cream eye shadow, then setting with a similarly toned powder eye shadow.

• Using a cream blush, then setting with a similarly toned powder blush. (See page 82.)

• Using a lovely, dewy foundation or tinted moisturiser and setting with a gentle dusting of translucent powder, just on the areas that are likely to get shiny.

But generally? Go for texture uniformity.

# NEVER, EVER FORGET WHICH SHADE OF MAKEUP YOU LOVE.

**PROBLEM:**

Too often my favourite makeup products rumble and romp around in the bottom of my handbag and, then, when they are on their last legs, I can't tell which shade it is, because the label, sticker or enamel has disappeared.

**SOLUTION:**

As soon as I know I have fallen for a product, especially those in the foundation or concealer realm, I pop down the shade number or name on a note in my phone, imaginatively titled MAKEUP SHADES. I used to simply write it down on a Scrap of Paper, but we all know where Scraps of Paper end up, and it's the same place as bobby pins and 50% of all socks.

**BONUS BIT OF AWESOMENESS:**

This is also very helpful when Significant Others or Lovely Friends go overseas and you want them to buy you something, because you can tell them the brand and shade/number and they have NO EXCUSE not to buy it for you unless they're naughty and get home and pretend the store was closed when they got there, but really they were too busy buying t-shirts from Zara to remember your one, minuscule, teeny request. *Why are you even friends with this person?*

*Bonus trick!*
*If you have paler skin, stick more to silver-pearl-toned makeup; if you have olive or darker skin, go more golden.*

# INSTANT REMEDIES.

**One**
If you've finished your makeup and all that powder and foundation and blush and bronzer is looking flat and heavy, rub some face cream between your hands and gently press it onto your face, which will inject some freshyness.

**Two**
Cheat the flawless, TV-ready, airbrushed look by dotting liquid foundation onto your chin, cheeks, forehead and a teeny bit on your schnoz. Now take a fluffy blush brush (a clean one) and with circular, buffing motions, blend your foundation over your face.

**Three**
Many makeup artists backstage at fashion week mist the models' faces with a hydrating spray *before* applying foundation (to give the skin some slip) and then *after* the makeup is complete. It gives vitamins and minerals and hydration and that delightful dewy, fresh-from-the-forest look.

# A WORD ON MINERAL MAKEUP.

And that word is: **caution**.

Mineral makeup (makeup made of several finely ground minerals, and usually but not always excluding talc, parabens and synthetics) is very popular for those with sensitive skin, or acne, or who have just had some sort of procedure (like a peel or botox or having a unicorn horn attached), but if you are after a flawless makeup finish, go easy with minerals.

I know! How outrageous. But as Oscars Makeup Genius Bruce Grayson once told me, 'It's unanimous that makeup artists don't like mineral makeup.'

Bruce says it's because it accentuates flaws. Y'see, women are encouraged to layer upon layer, and buff it in, and *then* add mineral blush, bronzer and shadow on top of that, which leads to the kind of texture, weight and shimmer that looks good on no one. And if you have problem skin, you definitely don't want to shimmer, because all THAT does is draw attention to flaws (see page 76).

'But problem skin is one of the big reasons women veer to minerals,' you cry, pounding the desk with your fist in a vulgar fashion.

True.

However, you can always switch to liquid mineral products, which have a more powder/matte finish. Try Napoleon Perdis' Advanced Mineral Makeup, or Jane Iredale Liquid Minerals A Foundation.

*Fun tip!*
Bruce loves using Aquaphor on celebs wearing long-last lipstick to 'reactivate' it.

# THE ONE MINUTE RULES: KNOW THEM AND ALWAYS, ALWAYS FOLLOW THEM. (IF YOU FEEL LIKE IT.)

Look, they're not *crucial*, in the same way you need to eat food at least once a week to stay alive, but they sure do make a whopping great difference to how your makeup sits for the day.

**Leave a minute in between applying your moisturiser and your primer.** This allows the moisturiser ingredients to sink in and do their thing before you slap on a layer of silicone.

**Leave a minute in between applying your primer and your foundation.** This allows the primer to spread evenly and settle into all the little cracks of your face and therefore create a flawless canvas before you put on your foundation.

**Leave a minute in between applying your eye cream and your under-eye concealer.** This allows the eye cream to sink in fully so that your concealer doesn't merge with it and, within an hour, either migrate up into your eye (dude! *grooooooss*) or crepe (little lines) with the overload of being put onto a surface that wasn't yet fully dry.

**Leave a minute in between applying your foundation and your blush or bronzer.** This allows the foundation to dry properly, so that your cheek products don't get stuck on the first piece of face you swipe the brush onto, or fail to blend and sit on top of your skin, rather than blending seamlessly into it.

*Bonus trick!*
For flawless application of a powder foundation, definitely let your moisturiser fully absorb before applying, otherwise your coverage will be all patchy.

I use the lags between to do fun things like curling eyelashes, and brushing teeth, and knitting small jumpers for baby possums.

89

# FIVE

## Makeup errors doing you zero favours.

### 1.

**Using a dark shade of foundation to appear more tanned.** Clever makeup artist-y types might disagree (they're much more talented than us at everything so we forgive them), but I say nay. Foundation exists to match and even out skin tone, and to conceal imperfections and create a uniform canvas for colour cosmetics.

By using a shade too dark for your skin, you risk looking muddy and the benefits above are void. Why not either apply some facial self-tanner (like Eco Tan Face Tan Water) before bed, or utilise bronzer on the points of the face where the sun would naturally hit, should you be you silly enough to let it. As per page 73, I think liquid or gel bronzers are the most subtle and 'skin-like' when buffed in gently with a fluffy blush brush. Set with a translucent powder or a soft wash of powder bronzer.

### 2.

**Going overboard with luminisers.** Glowing skin is a beacon for wide-eyed, envious compliments and a sign of buoyant health. And if you're crafty, you'll fake all of this with luminisers. The risk is in the application – thinking that more is better, because more gleaming skin = even *more* proof of great skin. But this is as wrong as Crocs with socks.

Illuminating products work best when applied subtly and sparingly: lightly underneath your foundation as an illuminating base, or a teeny bit mixed in with your liquid foundation, or as a finishing touch just on the high points of the cheekbones. Otherwise they start rebelling and making your skin look WORSE: visible pores, exacerbated fine lines and wrinkles, and highlighted blemishes. So, go easy, cowboy. (Lovely horse, by the way.)

**3.**

**Too much eye makeup during the day.**
Despite what the Kardashian/Jenners will have you think, heavily smoked-up eyes are pretty dramatic, and probably better for night-time, rather than being wasted under fluorescent office lighting or dropping down onto your cheeks as you take little Dwayne and Beryl to the park.

One way to indulge your love of kohl and shadow while keeping it daytime-appropriate is by sticking to top lash line and eyelid only, which will keep it fresh, or switching to brown.

**4.**

**All the hair product at the roots.** Aside from root lift sprays (and lightweight volume mousses), *most* hair styling products are best kept off the scalp, because they just make your hair greasier faster, which means more washing, which, der, sucks. Instead, apply from a few inches down. Even volume powder and dry shampoo can be applied just off the scalp. If you're a fine-haired kitten, same goes for your conditioner – apply from the mid-lengths to the ends only (if at all: conditioner isn't required at all on some hair types. Try skipping it and see! Outrageous!)

**5.**

**Applying lipstick straight from the bullet.** It's an inaccurate art, and often leads to feathering and error. Of course, if you're on the go, touching up with a quick *push* of lipstick (rather than swiping) onto the lips is fine, but there's a tremendous pay-off in lining the lips thoroughly, then using a lip brush to apply your lipstick. This will help with longevity, but also the look is much crisper, and the room for error much smaller, and the chance of being mistaken for Rihanna much higher.

# BEAUTY IS THE BEST WAY TO SNEAK INTO FANCY HIGH FASH BRANDS.

A lady cannot always ('never') afford a YSL tuxedo or Gucci heels or a Dior bag, but a lady *does* have a decent chance of procuring a beautiful YSL lipstick to slide out of her handbag after lunch, or of misting a Balenciaga scent on her person before she leaves the house, or of pulling out a Tom Ford bronzer in the bathroom to dazzle friends and strangers alike.

And well she should! Not only are these products of excellent quality, but designer cosmetics provide us with an accessible, glorious avenue into the luxury and elegance of a brand we would ordinarily be excluded from.

You don't need many of these special items; one or two is plenty. Just ask anyone who gets their hands on a new-season Chanel nail lacquer – the conversational currency and elevated social standing among girlfriends is brainbending! Add a Chanel lip gloss and a lady is set

for many months of delight when she paints her nails
or adorns her lips.

Now, you might be thinking, sixty-five CLAMS for a
LIPSTICK? Is this girl having a LAUGH? That's more
than my WHOLE OUTFIT cost! And almost as much
as my daily LOBSTER LINGUINE! And so on!

But as I explained up above, these are *luxury* items. They
are not everyday beauty items, thrashed and stashed in
your filthy little makeup bag; they are special and fancy,
deserving of a place on your bathroom sink next to a
candle or a small vase with a single rose in it: they are
social-media gold.

They will look good, and they will last, and they will
feel absolutely magnificent when applied in public. And
sometimes, that's all a lady wants. A bit of admiration
from some strangers for her fancy lipstick.

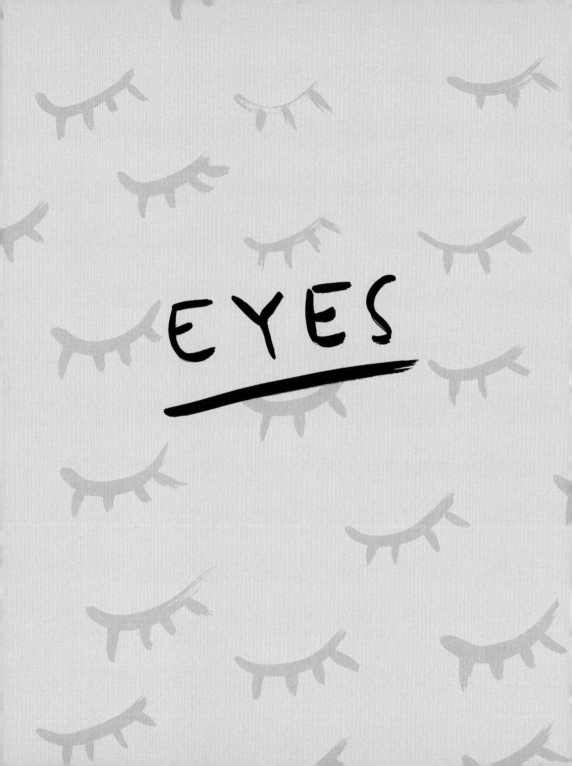

EYES

'Eyes, eyes, the magical face surprise,
like jewels in a diamond just sitting by,
waiting for some liner or mascara to wander by,
How will you dress up your eyes?' *

The eyes allow you to change your entire
look more than any other area of beauty.

Except for maybe the lips.

Oh, and hair.

And I guess a spray-tan can
make a heck of a difference too.

# AS MAGNETS CONSTANTLY PROVE: OPPOSITES ATTRACT.

**When it comes to the best and most flattering eye shadow for eye colour combinations, there is a simple rule:** Don't eat chicken that has been out of the fridge for 12 hours.

**Also there is this one, which is more relevant:** Use the opposite colour to your eye colour.

**Green eyes**
Plums, purples and lilacs.

**Options:** Stila Eye Shadow Trio in Venus, Covergirl Smoky Shadow Blast in Purple Plum, NARS Eyeshadow Duo in Charade.

**Blue eyes**
Browns, coppers and bronze.

**Options:** MAC Paint Pot in Constructivist, YSL Couture Palette in Afrique 3, Maybelline Eye Studio in Tough As Taupe.

**Hazel?**
Lucky you, you can wear anything the greenies or brownies do!

**Brown eyes**
Deep cobalt blue, baby blue and emerald green.

**Options:** Max Factor Masterpiece Colour Precision Eyeshadow in Stardust, Revlon Matte Eyeshadow in Riviera, Chanel Ombres Contraste Duo in Bleu-Tendre.

*Note:*

*Don't think it needs to be a full eyelid of shadow. Oh gosh, no! Even a swipe of liner or mascara in these tones does the trick. When it comes to coloured eye shadow, subtlety is always on the menu, and sometimes it tastes better than the degustation.*

# SAME, SAME BUT DEEPER.

**WHAT WE KNOW:**

- Green eyes pop most with purple tones.

- Blue eyes pop most with coppers, bronzes, browns.

- Brown eyes pop most with blues, purples, browns . . . anything, really. Lucky little squids.

**WHAT WE MAY NOT:**

- There is a fun little trick with eye shadow that directly contrasts with this, uh, contrast rule. And that is that wearing the same colour, but in a slightly deeper shade than your iris colour, is also very flattering.

- If you're using the exact same colour as your iris colour, go for an all-over wash of gentle shadow, or just use the shade as a liner. (Generally, the brighter the shadow, the less surface area you cover. Drag queens may argue this point.)

# WHY NOT CHOOSE YOUR EYE SHADOW ACCORDING TO YOUR HAIR COLOUR? COULD BE FUN, YOU KNOW...

It's very make-sensey to choose eye shadows that will complement and bring out your eye colour, but what say we shake things up a little by matching your **eye makeup to your hair colour** instead?

Try it and you will see instant glamour and allure!

**Blonde?** Sandstone, sand, cream and taupes.

**Brunette?** Latte, mocha and chocolate brown.

**Redhead?** Shades of copper, peach, brick-reds and browns or cool tones like pinks and lavenders.

**Grey hair?** Shades of greys, soft purples and gentle blues.

**Green hair?** Less swimming in chlorinated pools.

*Bonus trick!*

For an eye-shadow job with some kapow, use three shades from the same colour family (e.g. lilac, purple and dark plum). Gently apply the lightest colour over the entire eyelid, the medium shade up until the crease, and the darkest colour along the lash line.

*Bonus trick!*

If you're doing a natural, taupe shadow, add a touch of the most contrasting shadow colour for your iris colour in the outer corner of your eyelid.

# THERE ARE AROUND 327380 DIFFERENT WAYS TO DO A SMOKY EYE.

I *would* detail them all here, but the book has already gone to the printers now so sadly I cannot. However, I managed to get these ones done before all of that happened. *Phew!*

**Use chocolate tones instead of black and grey.** It makes for a softer, more seductive smoky and is more flattering than grey (but can be just as theatrical and intense, if that's a concern). Switching to brown is remarkably flattering if one has green, blue or brown eyes. That's right. *All of you.*

**Use plum liner and mauve shadow.** This is terrifically flattering on green eyes and is softer than blacks and charcoals. Smoke it up a little more than you would with your usual colours to get the same intensity, or keep it deliberately subtle (and closer to the lash line).

**Be careful using blues.** They can make it look as though you have under-eye circles, and tend to smudge and fade over the night and need constant re-application.

**Inject copper and bronze.** The perfect accompaniment to a brown-based smoky is a lid brimming with gilded metallics in warm copper and bronze tones. It looks astonishing on warm skin tones and flatters all eye colours.

**Go lighter on the top and move more to the bottom.** Instead of spending all your application time blending on the eyelid, take a smudging brush and blend charcoal or chocolate brown along and under the bottom lash line, to the point where you feel like a bit of a junkie. Trust me. It's so fashion, babe.

**Substitute browns and blacks for an intriguing gilded olive green.** Employing deep green as the principal colour is a devastatingly simple way to inject excitement into your smoky eye. Particularly enchanting on green eyes. (Try Urban Decay Moondust Eyeshadow in Zodiac.)

**Create layers of gun-metal grey and smoke.** Begin with a cream shadow in a menacing metallic grey all over the lid and build up the drama with subtly shimmering charcoals, blending out from the lash line up to the crease. Finish with strong black liner along the top and bottom lash line, and a stiff drink.

# A SIMPLE AND FAST SMOKY EYE THAT SUITS US ALL.

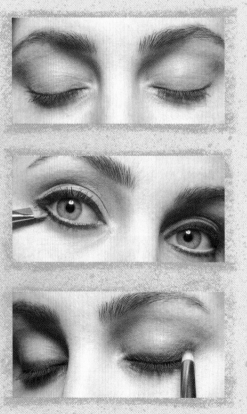

1 Apply concealer to the eyelid (not the whole face, just the eyelid) for a smooth canvas. (Of course, use a specific eye base/primer if you own one.)

2 Apply gel liner along the upper and lower lash lines as an eyeliner base. Do this with a thin, fine, angled liner brush – these are better than very thin, pointed brushes for those who aren't super-awesome at liner application. (Try the Body Shop's Slanted Brush.)

3 Use a brown eye shadow applied with a defining pencil brush on top of the eyelid liner to make it more dramatic, and to set the liner in place. This is a KEY makeup artist trick that you should definitely steal.

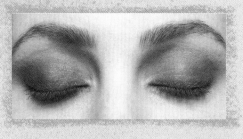

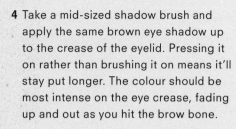

**4** Take a mid-sized shadow brush and apply the same brown eye shadow up to the crease of the eyelid. Pressing it on rather than brushing it on means it'll stay put longer. The colour should be most intense on the eye crease, fading up and out as you hit the brow bone.

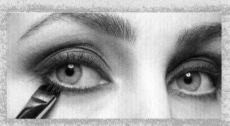

**5** Take a smudger brush (NARS does a great one) and some brown shadow and 'push-and-wiggle' underneath and into the lower lash line to make a sexy, soft, elongated smoky effect.

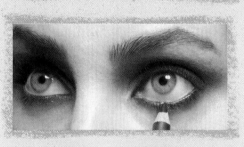

**6** Run black kohl along the inner and lower waterline of the eye (see page 108), then some brown kohl on top to further define the eye. Go as dark and intense as you wish.

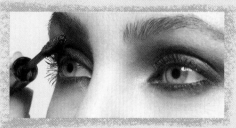

**7** Coat top lashes in black mascara. Many times. Do bottom lashes lightly if you wish.

**8** Apply your foundation to the rest of your face as normal. (Yes, eye makeup *before* foundation. Is common with smoky eyes. Means you don't have to reapply foundation if eye shadow falls down below the eye. See page 129.)

**9** Watch in awe as masses of sex appeal suddenly fly in from above.

# LOOSE EYE SHADOW IS MARVELLOUS WHEN APPLIED CORRECTLY.

*Bonus trick!*
Keep bright eye-shadow shades modern with black liner and mascara. MAC Eye Kohl in Smolder is a classic black eyeliner for super-fast smudgy sexy eyes.

*Bonus trick!*
There's usually enough shadow in the lid to use, and it means less mess.

If you're anything like me, you house an inner magpie. This magpie is drawn to shiny things and bright colours, and is the reason you accidentally buy sparkly, dangly necklaces and canary-yellow coin purses. And shimmering loose eye shadow. For example, MAC Pigment, which looks spectacular, especially when blended softly over the socket with a tear-shaped blending brush (I love Estée Lauder's).

The thing about loose eye shadow is that the less you use, the more elegant the effect. These shadows contain so much pigment that you really don't need much at all. Start by priming the eye so it has something to stick to – shadow primer or cream shadow are best. Use a stubby pencil shadow brush to push the powder onto the eyelid, always tapping off all the excess on your wrist first so you have only the most teeny amount to work with. Then, using your large blending brush, go back and forth over the eyelid like a windscreen wiper, blending the shadow ever so softly over the eyelid.

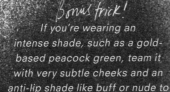

*Bonus trick!*
If you're wearing an intense shade, such as a gold-based peacock green, team it with very subtle cheeks and an anti-lip shade like buff or nude to keep the look from screaming up to Groovy on the Discometer.

*Bonus trick!*
You can also use loose shadow wet, in a technique called foiling. Just add a couple of drops of water – or better yet – saline eye drops to a dense shadow brush (or spongy shadow applicator – like the type that comes with eye shadow when you buy it) so it's damp, then press the brush into the lid of your loose powder and apply to the eyelid, patting it on and building up the intensity as desired. Sparkly! Dense! Intense! Magpie-riffic!

**Some loose shadow suggestions:**

• A subtly shimmery nude-champagne shade over the lid (try MAC Pigment in Naked or Maybelline NY Colour Tattoo Loose Powder in Barely Brazen), with black liner wings.

• A soft lilac shade over the whole lid, teamed with soft pink lipstick for a pretty, girly look.

• A deep violet shade in place of dull charcoal or brown for a dangerous and alluring take on the traditional smoky eye. Team with black liner and nude lipstick.

• A coppery, bronze shade with black liner, lots of bronzer and a nude lip in an effort at being a Latina Fox, à la Jenny Lopez or Jessy Alba.

• A plum, olive green or demure grey on the socket only, nice and neat, with a ladylike rose blush and a pink gloss or lipstick.

• The key is to keep things balanced, and always start with a light-handed approach.

# MAKE YOUR EYES APPEAR MORE OPEN AND BEAUTIFUL WITH HIGHLIGHTER.

Often when I have my makeup done professionally, the Makeup Artist Genius Type doing it will dab a little bit of highlighter (usually a shimmery, metallic or cream-coloured eye shadow or pencil) in the inner corners of my eyes (pretend technical term: inner 'V'). It makes me look wide-awake, as if my eyes are bigger and wider apart, and as if I am way prettier than I am.

Makeup artists do this because highlighter in these areas greedily snatches any available light and makes eyes look wider and more open. Which I think you'll agree is nice of them.

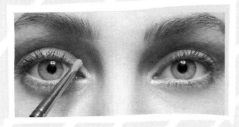 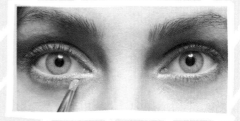

## NOW YOU DO IT!

- Before you place the highlighter in the inner corner of your eye, clean out any eye poo from the area.

- After you have done the rest of your eye shadow but before mascara: take a gold, bronze or peach-cream (avoid white – too harsh – and silver – rarely flattering) highlighting pencil, eye shadow or metallic cream shadow and draw a horizontal 'V' shape that follows the inner corner of your eye from top to bottom.

- If you're using shadow, use a pointed eyeliner brush (like MAC #219 Pencil Brush) for perfect application. Also, those little (otherwise pretty useless) applicators that come with eye shadow are good for this inner V work. Be wary when using loose shadows as they tend to get bored with staying in one place and start creeping down under the eye.

- Once you've applied, clean up any spill-down from the highlighter with a clean cotton tip.

**These are good:** BECCA Shimmering Skin Perfector Pressed in Opal, Kiko Perfect Eyes Duo Highlighter Pencil, Lancôme Color Design Eyeshadow in Gaze, L'Oréal Infallible Eyeshadow in Hourglass Beige, Too Faced Candlelight Glow Highlighting Powder Duo.

# MAKEUP SORCERY! USING EYE SHADOW AS EYELINER.

Using liquid liner pisses 100% of women off, and frustrates the rest. So flip that fiddly little pen/brush thing the bird and switch to using a wet eye shadow with an angled brush. It's faster, cheatier and easier for schmucks like me who hate liquid liner because they can't apply it very well.

## YOU'LL NEED:

• A fine, angled liner brush (they are crucial for good liner application – try Laura Mercier's Flat Eye Liner Brush, MAC's 266 Small Angle Brush or Napoleon Perdis' Angle Brush g5)

• Some water

• An eye shadow that is able to be used wet or dry*

• A hand

• Some eyelids

*Regarding the actual shadow: Test your eye shadows to see if they are going to work as liner by dipping your liner brush into water, then into your eye shadow. If the water makes the pigment disappear on your brush and it's too watery and sheer, or the water just sits on top of the shadow and won't blend, or the shadow won't sit on your skin properly, or build in intensity, give up. This is clearly not a wet/dry shadow.

**NEXT:**

Trot off and buy a couple of wet/dry shadows. The good-quality, finely milled variety, which are high in pigment, are best. A lot of brands kindly specify whether they're wet/dry, but I know, for example, that most NARS, Lancôme, Stila, Physicians Formula, Chanel, Bobbi Brown and Estée Lauder shadows are wet/dry. Make a habit of asking this question when you buy your eye shadow because I've seen too many marvellous makeup artists do this liner trick to know that it's worth finding out, and that wet/dry shadow is better than the non wet/dry variety. After all, you will be getting two products in one, you dingus!

**To do the actual trick:** Go to page 110.

A safe and flattering bet is always a soft, medium brown but here are some colour-combinations to make your iris colour stand out and make people gasp with delight:

**Blue eyes:** Gold, bronze, copper or any variant of brown.

**Green:** Olive green, purple or plum.

**Brown:** Peacock blue, baby blue or violet.

# WATERLINE AND DAZZLE EVERYONE!

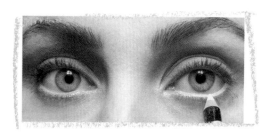

Putting eyeliner along that little strip of skin between the eyeball and your eyelashes can make *such a difference*, and create very different looks than what you might be used to. When you do it along the inner **lower lash line**, encompassing the bottom of your eye, it's called **waterlining**.

Depending on what you apply here, you can really open up the eye and make it look bigger, or you can make it look very rock and roll indeed (but sometimes smaller).

**Make the eyes look bigger:** Use a fleshy-pinky-white toned eye pencil. This counters redness and really wakes everything the heck up. I love MAC's Chromographic pencil for this.

**Make the eyes look night-time and sexy:** Use black pencil, preferably waterproof. But a warning: going the entire way along can make your eye look smaller than it is, and it's harsher too. I usually just line the outer third for a feline look, and then smudge some liner and eye shadow into the lash line for extra SCHWING. (CoverGirl's Liquiline Blast is ideal.)

For some reason a jet-black waterline is especially popular with the very young (sassy teens going batshit crazy with black kohl to look older) or the very old (dames who need to put the liner down cos it is not only doing them no favours, it is actually stealing favours from them as they slumber) but that does not mean it should be. Use with caution.

# TIGHTLINE AND DAZZLE EVEN MORE!

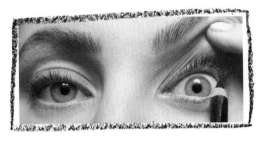

When you **do it on the top**, along that line that is closest to your actual eyeball and upper lash line, it's called **tightlining**. (Probably cos it's so damn tight getting in there, amirite ladies???)

You should stick to black, brown or a dark colour up here, and a pencil liner is the way to go.

I prefer tightlining to applying liner on top of the lash line (the lid line) because it emphasises the lashes, opens up the eyes (liner on top of the lid can appear to close your eyes because it creates a severe outline), makes your eyes look whiter and brighter and prettier without any smooshing or running of eyeliner up and over the eyelid. Also, it makes a smoky eye (see page 100) look *phenomenal*.

*Remember:*
*Whether you're tightlining or waterlining, keep the pinky in place for a few moments after applying the liner so it can set.*

# THE CHEAT'S WAY TO DO CLASSIC LIQUID LINER.

1 Apply concealer or eyelid primer over the lid, then apply a nude, neutral shadow over your eyelid, or even just some loose powder. This hides veins and gives the eyes a fresher, open look.

2 Take an angled, flat liner brush and dip it into water.

3 Now take the wet brush and dip it into black or brown eye shadow. (See page 106 to ensure you're using one that will work.) This is your 'practice' liner line.

4 Take the brush very carefully along your entire lash line, trying to keep the line half on your lashes and half on your eyelid so that it's not an obvious line – this boosts your lashes and makes them fatter. There shouldn't be any skin showing between the line and your lashes. Dab on bit by bit if it's easier than one fluid line.

5 Stop at the end of your lash line, or take the brush and kick it up into a little 'wing' around ½ cm before you get to the end. (The angle you want is the one you'd get if you were applying liner to your lower lash line and kept going up . . .) (Alternatively, see page 112 for a cheat on this. Because look, I'll be honest: it's hard.)

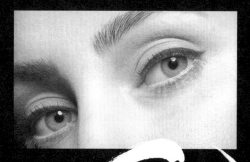

**6** Go over the line a few times to make sure it's neat, or if you want more colour.

**7** Once you're happy with the line, take your brush and pop the tiniest amount of gel or creamy liner on both sides of it. Using one of these liners is key: they're quick to dry, look crisp but soft and are very long-lasting. (Try Clinique, MAC, Bobbi Brown, Laura Mercier.) Using the liner, very carefully follow the line you made with your shadow, including the wing if you did one.

**8** Apply two coats of mascara.

**9** Wink cutely at yourself.

*Bonus trick!*

*Keep Very Shimmery or Exciting Eye Shadows modern and less ridiculous by using them as a liner instead. Apply them with a wet, flat brush. You may have to keep wetting the brush, but this will make the colour last forever. And one day after that.*

# USE CUNNING WIZARDRY TO CHEAT YOUR WAY INTO WINGED LINER.

This trick certainly changed the way I do my makeup, in an 'I could never do winged liner before but now I can' kind of way. It's clever because it relies on *removing and cleaning up what ISN'T the wing, rather than creating what IS the wing.* I like that brand of topsy-turvy, lateral thinking. (It's why I prefer to pour milk into the Milo tin, instead of the more common Milo-into-milk technique.)

There's no perfect angles, no super-accurate and precise liner application, and no impossible mirror positioning required. And yet you will create those sexy, feline Angie Jolie liner wings. Imagine *that*. Or better still, do it.

**The best kind of concealer for this purpose:** is thick and creamy. It needs to give good coverage, but be paint-able, and build-able without caking and looking too obvious. I like Laura Mercier Secret Concealer, or blending a touch of foundation (for added 'paintability') with NARS Radiant Creamy Concealer.

**The best kind of concealer brush for this purpose:** is one that will give you precise application, is firm and flat and is made of synthetic hair – these are best for blending liquid and cream makeup because they don't absorb as much product as natural-hair brushes. (I use a second concealer brush for applying cream shadow. How about that!) I like the Benefit Concealer Brush for this trick.

**When you have them both:**

1 This trick works on makeup you have already applied. If you haven't yet applied any eye makeup, apply eye shadow over the eyelid and liner along the lash line as normal, but take it out past the end of the lash line, so that you have an area to 'clean up'. Of course, you can just use liner if you prefer. (Take it out further than normal and fatten it up to enjoy more scope with your concealer angle.) I've found this trick to work with shadow, gel, pencil and liquid liner, although the more 'stay-put' liners should be worked on before they are totally dry.

*Or you could do this:*

*For a beautifully defined upper lash line with a natural look, gently dot the lash line with an eyeliner pencil (go for a soft waxy one rather than the old-school pointy ones) and then blend into the lashes with a cotton tip. This makes your lashes appear thicker and more delicious without looking like you're wearing a dollop of liner.*

**2** Taking your concealer brush dipped in concealer 'paint', begin concealing under the eye area as usual, starting at the inner corner and going along under the eye. Then start to take it up in a wing at the outer corner, following the natural line of the lower lash line, upwards. Use one clean stroke if possible.

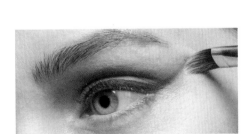

**3** Keep going up, all the way to past your eyebrow (or even further – you want all the shadow and liner on the outside of your 'line' to be cleaned away/ concealed), following that same sharp angle. Go over it a few times and pat the concealer (*not on the line* – keep that sharp; pat underneath only) into your skin so it blends into your skin tone and there is no obvious concealer patch. Gently glide your middle finger along the wing for a final clean-up. Cheatastic.

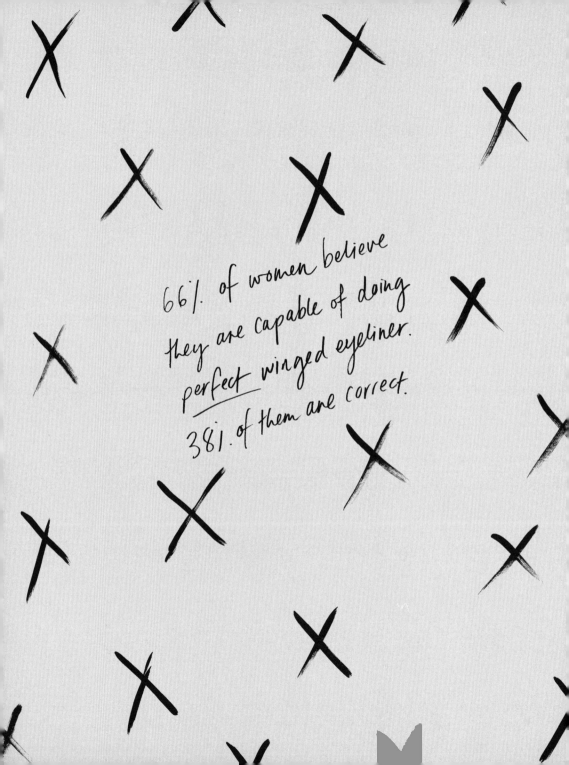

66% of women believe they are capable of doing _perfect_ winged eyeliner.

38% of them are correct.

# THERE IS A MUCH EASIER WAY TO REMOVE EYE MAKEUP.

**What I will be mentioning on this page:**
That you need **eye makeup remover pads** in your life.
I like the Almay ones. (Don't buy the oily ones; the oil
gets in your eyes and it's annoying. Stay oil-free.) These
are round cottony pads doused in remover and they will
decrease your eye-makeup removal time and energy by
up to 675%.

As someone who often Wears Too Much Eye Makeup
Because It Is Fun and Also Her Job, Kind Of, I find eye
makeup remover pads marvellous for removing stubborn
eyeliner and smoky-eye-ness and that thing
I tried to pull off that I saw in *Vogue* magazine where
the girl had red glitter everywhere, except that it looked
terrific on her, probably because she is a model and a
makeup artist did hers.

But I digress. All you do is press a pad on each closed
eye for 10 seconds and then gently wipe down and off.
It'll take a few wipes – be gentle, please – but it'll all go,
and then when you wash your face, even the sneakiest
bits of leftover mascara and liner will be forced to shove
off, and all you will be left with are your pretty, clean
little eyelets. (See page 130 for more.)

**What I will not be mentioning on this page:**
That I definitely have a snail trail. I do. I pretend
I don't but I definitely do.

# INSTANTLY MAKE YOUR EYES LOOK BIGGER.

The sad truth about eye makeup is that sometimes it hates us and deliberately makes perfectly lovely-sized eyes look small and beady.

**HOW TO ENSURE THIS DOESN'T HAPPEN TO YOU:**

1 Use two eyeliners. One should be a pink-fleshy-white highlighter (see page 108), and one should be a darker matte colour (like Estée Lauder's Double Wear Stay-in-Place Eye Pencil in Coffee, which flatters *everyone*).

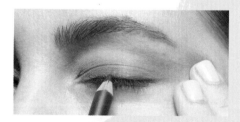

2 Take the dark pencil and dot between the upper lashes. Now do the lower lashes, but do the dotting business ONLY in the middle of the lower lash line, under the pupil.

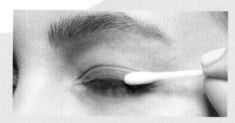

3 Use a smudger brush (or cotton tip) to gently smudge in the liner.

**4** Next, take the highlighter pencil and waterline (see page 108 to find out what the heck this is, how to do it and why you must learn) both the top and bottom of the eye.

**5** Now, connect the two highlighted lines at the outer corner of the eye.

**ANOTHER WAY TO ENSURE IT:**
Never use black liner on the waterline.

Well. Look at you, big eyes! Probably get confused with a baby cow with those walloping great googlers.

# USE MANY MASCARA FORMULAS ALL AT ONCE FOR THE MOST IMPRESSIVE LASHES ON EARTH (AND MARS).

Get prescriptive with your lashes. Think of them as a patient needing the correct medication to get them to their optimal state.

What do they lack? What do they need? What are your lashiest desires? How do they look in that dream where that total hunk from the coffee shop falls in love with you over gluten-free toasted banana bread with no butter?

You may already have curly lashes and only want length and volume. Or you may have long lashes that don't need lengthening.

Choose your wish list and then choose a flock of mascaras to facilitate it. At the very least, use two different formulas of mascara.

*Bonus trick!*

*Coloured mascara? Why not, you creative little crumpet! The best/least '80s way to use it is either to coat just the tips or your lashes, after applying regular black mascara, or to colour-match the mascara to your eye shadow.*

**HERE'S MY PRESCRIPTION, AS AN EXAMPLE. I HAVE SHORT, THIN LASHES AND WISH FOR THEM TO BE THE OPPOSITE.**

1 Run a defining, comb-style mascara (like L'Oréal Paris Telescopic Mascara) through the lashes, from root to tip. This is the best kind of mascara to begin with in any prescription as it separates the lashes.

2 Run a lengthening mascara (like Benefit They're Real) through the lashes. Now I have definition and length but, being a greedy little salami, I wish for volume also.

3 Finish with a coat from a big, fat volume builder (like CoverGirl Lashblast Volume Mascara). Really get in there at the root – wiggle the wand and then fan it out.

The final effect is simply dazzling. You may even find, after applying your prescriptive mascara routine, that it negates the need to wear false lashes! Imagine that.

*Bonus trick!*

*Apply each of the mascara coats gently and slowly on the lashes to prevent clumping, but don't let each layer get dry before applying the next. So go fast!...But go slow, too.*

*Trickier trick!*

*Try a lashlift for 'permanent' curl. It lasts around 6 weeks, includes a tint, and means your lash curler will be very bored indeed. I love lashlifts. Much.*

# FOR THOSE WHO INSIST ON WEARING BOTTOM-LASH MASCARA.

If you asked, 'Is mascara on the bottom lashes a do or a don't?', I would say: 'Are you crazy like a coconut?! It falls off, it sticks to your top lashes, from a distance it makes you look like you have dark circles, and it does the opposite of that pretty, open-eyed look you were after. DON'T! *It's a don't!'*

But then I learned A Trick, and suddenly I wasn't so anti-bottom-lash mascara (and politically incorrect regarding mentally unstable coconuts).

## Know this:

*If you bodge your mascara midway through the application, don't get all cranky and frustratey because you were supposed to be out the door three minutes ago; just wait till your mascara has dried completely, then take a cotton tip and lightly 'scratch' off the naughty mascara. Or use your fingernail like I do, even though I shouldn't encourage such things.*

## Bonus trick!

*Try a 'tubular' mascara if you're sick of smudging, drop-down, or hard-to-remove mascara. It requires no remover, only warm water. All you do is gently slide your thumb and index finger down your lashes, and the mascara comes off like little tubes. All in the shower, all in 10 seconds. I am fanatical about them – in particular, Clinique Lash Power Mascara and Kevyn Aucoin's Volume Mascara.*

**THE TRICK IS THIS:**

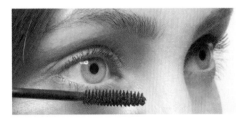

**1** Apply mascara to your top lashes as normal.

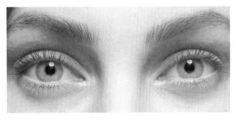

**3** Move the mascara wand gently around the bottom lashes and repeat the flutter a few times until they're all coated.

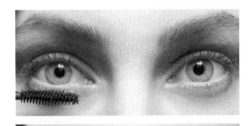

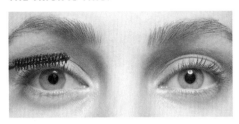

It's like a wee little stamp, see? And when you take away the wand, you have perfectly coated bottom lashes that are defined without being visibly coated in globs of mascara.

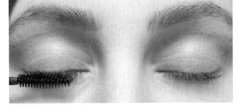

**2** Rest your wand/brush on your bottom lashes, right in at the roots, and flutter your eyes closed a few times.

# MASCARA FOR LONG, FEATHERY LASHED LADIES.

It's easy for a biased hack of a journalist with Mascara Length Deficit to write only on lengthening, curling, defining and volumising mascaras.

But that would be unfair to those with long, feathery, thick lashes who require information on products that will give their lashes **colour and style**, but not **length and volume**.

Yes, we resent them and their genetic mascara jackpot, but we must also pity them, for when the poor lambs purchase the latest razzle-dazz mascaras, they get dropdown: the entire eye area becomes cartoonesque and, within a few hours, the look is not dissimilar to that of a drag queen after a large night out revelling.

*And we can't have that.*

**If you have very long lashes,** steer clear of volume-boosting mascaras. They contain fibres to boost the fatness of the lashes and plump them up. This gives ol' stumpylashes here a chance, but will be nothing short of *horrific* for ladies who already have long eye curtains.

**If you have lots and lots and lots of lashes,** avoid lash-defining mascaras (like Chanel Inimitable and CoverGirl Lash Exact Mascara). The little rubber/silicone combs are BRILLIANT for the lash-deprived, but they exist to *bring out every single lash on your eye*, and when you have billions of lashlets, you may not want that.

**Go simple.** You don't want technological mastery and whistles and bells when you already have an impressive set of lashes. You just want some colour. So, have your lashes tinted, consider a lashlift for curl, and buy mascaras that trade on 'natural-looking lashes', like that lovable old tart, Maybelline Great Lash Mascara.

# MAKEUP ARTISTS WEEP INSIDE WHEN WE COMMONERS APPLY OUR MASCARA:

- on the underside of our lashes only
- from halfway up the lash
- sweeping directly up so that the lashes are stiff and vertical

**HERE ARE THEIR REASONS:**

**1** When you paint the tops of your lashes as well as the underside, they become thicker and give a flawless, defined look to anyone observing said lashes, should you ever blink.

**2** Applying your mascara from halfway up the lash creates a distinct line that is obvious to everyone who looks at you as you blink except for you because, sadly, as you're not able to see yourself when your eyes are closed; your mirror just can't help in this situation. This situation is especially pronounced when your mascara is a thick, volume-boosting variety and your lashes are thin, or you're a fair-headed minx.

**3** Vertical sweeping can make your lashes look unnatural because they usually have a slight curl and span out towards the outer corner of the eyelid. Wiggling at the base and then sweeping the wand/comb out gently to the side gives a prettier, wide-eyed look.

*Lashy tips!*

- *Only ever use your lash curler on mascara-free lashes, and do two clamps: one at the roots of the lash and one halfway up. Splash out and do three if you've got an extra eight seconds.*

- *Hold a teaspoon over the eyelid against the upper lash line and apply your mascara against it. Lashes will be treated to a little curl and there'll be no mascara errors on the eyelids.*

- *Lightly brush your lashes with your face powder before applying mascara. The powder and the mascara will form a paste to temporarily thicken your lashes. Marvellous!*

# REGARDING PUMPING YOUR MASCARA...

You know how when you want more mascara on the comb/wand, you pump the wand in and out of the tube?

No.

No.

*No.*

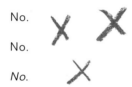

I don't know how many times you have to be told this, but we never, ever pump the mascara wand in and out of the tube.

Why? Because that naughty pumpy action forces air into the mascara formula, which oxidises it, which in turn breeds bacterial nasties that SO, DESPERATELY, want to give you the kind of gnarly infected eye that would see you wearing a non-ironic pirate patch for a few days.

**Do this instead:** Gently twist the wand around as you pull it out, and do the same when it goes back in. This will coat the wand with all the formula you need.

**But you know what? You really shouldn't even need to do that because:**

**1** Your mascara should get chucked after 10–12 weeks and if you're scraping the bottom, for the sake of stys* – please just buy a new one.

**2** Do you have ANY idea how much cash gets injected into making these wands and rims and tubes? Millions. Literally. Millions of dollars get spent in R&D making sure you never, ever need to do anything that even looks like pumping the wand, and that you have an enjoyable mascara experience in general and buy the very same one next time. Mascaras form the basis of many a cosmetic company's base fortune, which means that you will keep getting better mascaras, and the cosmetic company's CEO can afford to buy their children purebred puppies at Christmas, so everyone wins.

*No pumping!* No pumping. Make your mascara a pump-free zone.

*\*Sty? Gently rub a cotton tip dipped in baby shampoo over it, back and forth. It works!*

# THE THING ABOUT WATERPROOF MASCARA...

...is that, like death metal, it's just misunderstood.

**Great things about waterproof mascara:**
It's superb for those who want mascara on their bottom lashes but find their volume-building mascara is smudging and falling down.

It's excellent for people who may already be using a light mascara, but *still* find that they get dropdown, for whatever reason.

It's rad for summer. Because it's hot. And humid. And we sweat. And swim. And dance. And regular mascara can't always cope in such heady conditions.

**How to remove your waterproof mascara:**
With a cleansing oil (see page 19). The oil destroys the hardcore waterproofy bonds and the mascara comes off like a dream. Try Dermalogica PreCleanse, which also removes long-last makeup and sunscreens. The key is that you must use it on a dry face. Rub it on (even over your closed eyes) and massage it in, then add water and lather it off. Then cleanse as per normal.

It doesn't sting, it's very gentle and non-irritating and, well, it's just swell.

# THIS IS WHY YOUR MASCARA IS SMUDGING.

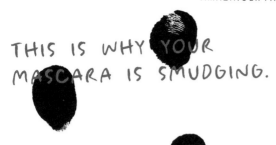

**FIRST, LET'S GET SOME THINGS STRAIGHT:**

- Waterproof does not automatically mean smudge-proof

- Your skin type ('oily'), type of lashes ('small', 'long', 'weak') and activity ('breakdancing') will influence smudge likeliness.

- Swipe your mascara wand with a tissue for excess before applying.

- Some mascara just smudges more than others.

- Do not use mascara on your bottom lashes if you get smudging a lot.

- Switch to a waterproof or gel liner instead of plain ol' kohl.

- Smudges make you look sloppy and tired. Forbid it.

- Smudges is a weird word if you say it too much.

**OKAY, GOOD. NOW, LET'S GET SOME THINGS BENDY:**

It might be cos your lashes can't handle the weight of the mascara you use. This is common when you have very fine lashes teamed with a deep passion for thick, volume-boosting mascaras (see page 116). The thing about these mascaras is that they use fibres to add thickness, and if your lashes are all wussy and weak (or too long, HAHAHA AS IF THERE IS SUCH A THING HAHAHA), they won't be able to withstand all that extra weight, so the mascara falls off. Try using a curling or lengthening mascara instead, or perhaps a 'natural-look' mascara (like Maybelline Full 'n Soft Mascara), or a simple defining mascara on top of a lash primer, which will give you both volume, definition and staying power. And probably the ability to sing in Spanish.

**Or** it could be cos you have oily skin, or too much eye cream/concealer around the eye, which is sneaking up into the lash line and making the mascara (and liner) bleed and smudge; the oils get up there and dissolve your mascara and break it down. (Think about it, this is why the best makeup removers are oil-based: oil is good at removing and dissolving makeup.) Try applying some blotting paper and then loose powder over your concealer/eye cream to stop it causing mischief, and a lash primer like MAC Prep + Prime Lash before your mascara.

**Or** *maybe* it's actually your liner causing mischief, not your mascara. Naughty liner! Giving mascara a filthy rep. I recommend a waterproof pencil liner on the lower lash line (like Make Up For Ever Aqua Eyes). Go for a gel liner along the top, like Stila Smudge Pot or MAC Fluidline, then set with powder eye shadow in the same colour. Your liner won't budge, bruh.

**Or** perhaps your mascara formula is the kind that smudges or flakes and then you rub your eyes – causing smudges. This is when I recommend waterproof mascara, or, even better, tubular (see page 120), which I wear religiously. They don't smudge, or run, even in severe humidity, sweat or during gentle, sweet sobbing, but they probably won't outlast full-blown ugly crying.

# LOOK YOUNGER REAL FAST.

Don't wear mascara.

I read this in an interview with Christy Turlington. She swore that the fastest way to look young and fresh was to Not Wear Mascara.

Now, I already drop the mascara on the weekends (weekday makeup is tricky; weekends are quicky) but I've started to stealthily drop it during the week too – not for lazy purposes, you understand, but for 'fresh' purposes.

**But! One must complement the lack of lashes (which on a lot of people can make them feel naked) by:**

• Not wearing any eye shadow

• Wearing a lovely, light-reflecting foundation or BB cream (the more radiant the better – fits in nicely with the whole healthy, fresh-faced thing)

• Wearing a light smattering of bronzer and/or a flush of cream blush on the cheeks

• Concealer in all the right places, especially under the eyes

• Curling the lashes to make the look into a 'fresh, youthful look as advised by a '90s supermodel' as opposed to an 'I forgot to wear mascara today' look, even tinting them if you can be bothered

• Mentally preparing for the annoyance of being asked for ID when you go to buy a slab of beer.

# FOUNDATION AFTER EYE MAKEUP. NO! REALLY?

I remember learning this trick 4000 years ago and being terribly perplexed: **Do your eye makeup first, then do your foundation and concealer.**

WHAT?! I thought in caps lock. BUT THAT GOES AGAINST EVERYTHING I'VE EVER BEEN TAUGHT ABOUT MAKEUP FROM THOSE OLDER GIRLS AT SCHOOL!

Which is the best reason to do it.

The more you unlearn amateur teenage makeup application, the better you will look.

**Here's the rub:** By doing your intricate eye shadow work *before* applying foundation (always prep the eyelids with some concealer and/or primer/cream shadow), you save all that cleaning up

and retouching that so often follows the Standard Application Method.

If you apply all your foundation and concealer first, and then some eye shadow falls down below the eye (as it inevitably does), you have to carefully remove it, then reapply your foundation and concealer – and very rarely does it look the same. Whereas if you're clean-skinned and some product falls down, you can easily clean it up without reapplying foundation or concealer.

Just like that new g-string bikini, this method just takes a little getting used to. But you'll see how much sense it makes when you do it. *Especially* if you're a fan of the smoky eye. (See page 96.)

# THE CORRECT WAY TO TREAT YOUR EYE AREA.

**No wipey wipey, ever.**
Feel that skin under your eye. Now. Do it now. Get your index fingy and actually feel it. GOSH it's thin, isn't it? Now feel your forehead/cheeks/chin/nose. Much thicker and bouncier, aren't they? That's because the skin around your eye is super delicate and needs to be that way so that your eyes can move around to look at handsome people surreptitiously, and because it is so fragile and special, it deserves some respect.

**When we apply eye cream, we don't go up any higher than the 'orbital bone', which is the bone that runs under the eye socket.** Due to body heat, anything you apply under your eyes will automatically migrate up. (This is also why eyeliner always runs down from the lower rim of your eye; the heat of your hot little body makes it melt.) Keeping this in mind, if you apply eye cream right up under your eye, guess where it's gonna be real soon? (Hint: Not Sweden.) The key is to keep your eye cream on that bone under your eye socket because it will automatically sneak its little way up towards your eye anyway.

**When we remove product from that region, we go gently, gently, so gently, and we never, ever drag or pull.** The skin around your eye has few, if any, oil glands. It can't 'bounce back' from wear and tear like the rest of your face can. It just stretches and stays that way. Which is how wrinkles form. So, for example, when you're removing eye makeup, hold the makeup remover pad (see page 115 for more about these) over the eye for 5–10 seconds, then gently drag it down your lashes towards the floor, rather than yanking it out to the side again and again.

**Tap tap, not rub rub.**
Tapping in your product with your rude finger (just go up and down the orbital bone a few times) is not only lovely and gentle, but it promotes circulation, which in turn does wonders for getting rid of dark circles and puffiness. Nice!

# DO YOU OWN AN EYE MASK?

*Fun tip!*
When you apply eye cream to puffy eyes, start dabbing it in right up on the nose, and continue along under the eye and out to the temples. These two spots are drainage areas, and it's no good tap-tap-tapping all along those bags of yours if all that puffiness has nowhere to drain out.

Not that little satin pillow thingy you wear at night, I mean an actual mask (like the ones we have for our face, from a tube or jar) for the eye area.

If you do not, may I sit you down and hold both your hands in mine and recommend changing this? Especially if you are a busy person, or a party person, or a have-a-young-baby person, or a can't-sleep person. The eye area is the first place fatigue shows, so investing in something to counter said fatigue makes sense. Wouldn't you agree?

('Investing' was the operative word. These aren't cheap.)

Popping one of these on for 10 minutes as you try to figure out how to work the kettle (or before a party) makes such a difference. And as a bonus, your concealer and illuminator will sit so, so smoothly.

1 The Sisley Eye Contour Mask has arnica (great for getting swelling/puffiness down) and really re-hydrates and smooths the eye area. I keep mine in the fridge. *Dulicious.*

2 The Gernetic Eye Mask boosts micro-circulation and the lymphatic drainage of the eye area and which you can IMMEDIATELY feel working on your circulation (bad circulation is the main cause of dark circles) because it tingles and brings the blood to the surface.

3 The SK-II Signs Eye Mask, two little 'stickers' that are always being used backstage on models pre-runway, works on fatigue and dehydration, but will also help with dark circles and fine lines and brighten up the whole dingin' area. They're also great when flying because of their disposable nature and lack of motion sickness.

# FIVE
## Fixes for beauty glitches.

I know everyone reading (and writing) this book looks utterly perfect all of the time, even when they have just finished rescuing small mud bears (they exist, look it up), but sometimes, sometimes we drop our incredibly perfect glossy veneer. How disgusting of us! Here are some snappy fixes should it ever happen again.
(I sure hope not.)

## 1.

**White gunk at the corners of your mouth.** Spit and lip product build-up at the corners of the mouth is gross. Sorry, but it is. It happens if you're talking a lot, and not drinking enough water or freshening up. It's my worst fear when I'm hosting events and people are staring at me as I chat for 45 minutes. (That, and earthquakes.) (And ferrets.) Your best chance of avoiding it is sipping water regularly, using a lip stain, matte lip pencil or crayon-style lip product all over the lips, and keeping any gloss or creamy lipstick to just the centre of your lips. Also, discreetly open wide and scrape the nails of your thumb and index finger around the outer sides of the lips every now and again just in case. Thanks, grosso.

## 2.

**Too much blush, bronzer or shimmer on the cheeks.** Take a foundation brush (or a sponge, or your fingers) and lightly paint some liquid foundation over the offending area, which will tone it down without removing all colour (MAC Studio Face and Body is perfect for this). Or take some mineral powder foundation and buff some over the top, just until you have muted the brightness or shimmer, or tempered the muddiness. You won't need to ('really shouldn't') add any more cheek product.

### 3.

**It's late in the day and you have a very crinkly, dry face, but no skin care.** Hand cream is a no-no, just before you telepathically ask. Instead, head to the kitchen, possums! That's where coconut/olive oil lives, and that's what you can lightly, using your index and middle fingers, press onto your face, especially around the crinkly parts, like the eyes. This will add glow and freshness. Even over your makeup, yes. (Self-raising flour, not so much.)

### 4.

**You have been crying. And wish to not show it.** If possible, use a cold compress on the area to calm swelling and puffiness. Then some redness or allergy-clearing eye drops. Makeup-wise, reapply corrector and concealer, then go for a navy or plum eyeliner instead of black (it will make your eyes look brighter) and waterline the lower lash line with a white or flesh-toned liner to brighten and open up the eyes. Lash curler and mascara (waterproof if you think you'll be crying again, although personally I think you're better off without him) and you're done.

### 5.

**You've applied too much perfume.** It's okay, Stinkarella, we can fix this. Either apply some basic, non-scented body lotion over the scented skin, or remove the fragrance from the skin (almost) altogether with a baby wipe. And in future, maybe just spritz into the air and walk through it.

# LATE NIGHT, HUH?

Like a 'nonchalant' text to a new lover, extra-dark circles demand extra attention.

**1** Put two teaspoons in the freezer before you shower.

**2** Moisturise your tired, sorry little face and press those spoons tight against the skin under both eyes for a few minutes.

**3** Pat on your eye cream like little airy-fairy pitter patter steps up and down your under-eye – the massage will help get the stagnant blood circulating.

**4** Or, use an eye mask specifically created to wallop dark circles (see page 131).

**5** Begin by patting on a pink- or peach-toned corrector. It's worth buying one of these if you often get dark circles – like a remote without a TV, concealer cannot do the job alone. I love Napoleon Perdis' The One Concealer.

**6** Apply your concealer, taking it right up onto the nose and right out to where the eyebrow finishes. Use a press and roll motion as that will layer the product by building up coverage. Sweeping motions will thin out the product.

**7** Finish with a creamy, liquid illuminator, doing that upside-down triangle trick on page 67.

# YOUR BROWS ARE MAKING YOU UGLY.

But you made them ugly first, so it's only fair. Of course, I don't mean 'you' personally, I mean the universal you, the 'You' that is from the same family as 'They' when we say things like, 'They say toads give you warts.' (See how that sentence cleverly used both the 'you' and the 'they'? It was an accident, to be honest, but I think we can all agree it was inspired.)

But back to bad brows. In particular, too-thin brows. Of which I am an expert, because I had them for 10 years. And they are *wrongo*.

Overly thin brows amplify flaws and make non-flaws start to become one. They make your nose look bigger. Chin pointier. Face wider. They make your features look harsher and sharper, and pull the face up in an unnaturally taut and severe manner. It's ageing and it's unflattering.

But with thicker, natural brows, the face appears balanced, younger, fresher. The eyes, cheeks and even the lips are enhanced. Think of your brows as a kind of photo frame around your features: no single feature stands out, but they all play along harmoniously, like a small troupe

of dancers with bells in the Spanish countryside, or AC/DC.

These days, my brows are thick and full, and after growing them out (*such* fun) I have them shaped and tinted every month so that they stay this way, and I am adamant that their thickness is maintained. But for some women, who have been plucking and waxing forever, or who were just born with thin or sparse brows, it's a bit trickier.

To these women I say: **tint**. Professional tinting (costs about 10–15 gold coins) will darken the brows, fill in the gaps and, if you go dark enough, create the illusion of thicker brows. (As a general rule, have your brows one to two shades darker than your hair colour.)

*Bonus tip!*
Taking sea-kelp supplements apparently aids hair growth. Which could be handy if you're trying to grow your brows out.

*Bonus tip!*
Lash and brow serums and conditioners improve the length, and thickness of the hair, and having used them myself, I reckon they do work. (I tried EyEnvy. Key is using it EVERY night.)

135

# Q: HOW DO I SHAPE MY BROWS PERFECTLY AT HOME?

**A:** You can't and you don't. You pay a professional to do it. Eyebrow shaping is NOT an area of DIY. No, no, no.

When locating said professional, always go by reputation and recommendation. If someone you know has exceptional-looking brows, ask her who does them. That's how we find these little brow-shaping masters, who quite often work from home in the suburbs and don't have so much as a business card, let alone a website or full-page advertisements in *Vogue*.

If you can't find your own special master, go to a department store and head to counters like Benefit, Estée Lauder, shu uemura, MAC or Bobbi Brown, which usually house brow-shaping experts.

*Bonus trick!*
*I prefer not to have my brows waxed (not precise enough), just tweezed and trimmed a touch. Threading is also great.*

136

**WHY BROW-SHAPING IS SO IMPORTANT:**

1 **Eyebrows are the most crucial element in shaping your face, and, well, whole appearance.** If shaped correctly, they flatter your face, balance out your features, make you look fresher and more youthful, and frame your eyes. Oh, sure, you laugh now, but next time you see a woman with over-plucked, over-arched, awful eyebrows, tell me you're able to focus on her lovely eyes or cheekbones over those brows. You can't. Impossible. In the symphony that is the face, bad brows are the off-key tuba.

2 **Your eyebrows must flatter your face shape.** That might mean keeping them quite straight, if you have a long face. Or, for an oval face, creating more of an arch. It's quite mathematical, and something best left to a pro. So leave it to a pro.

3 **The shape and grooming of your eyebrows can make your eyes look bigger, and open up your face.** A pair of brows with a perfect shape and a tint (or beautifully filled-in) means you can wear less makeup, have more hangovers, and get less botox. Not even kidding.

4 **To spend 50 clams on making your face as spatially balanced, youthful and alluring as possible makes sense.** Spending that amount on a mani or pedi, which you can do yourself and is over in two weeks, doesn't. Spend it on the brows. Even if you can only afford to go once, *go once*. Get the template set, then tweeze strays until you can afford to go back again.

# HOW TO TWEEZE YOUR BROWS BETWEEN SHAPING APPOINTMENTS*.

1 Have a shower or bath – this loosens up the hair and makes tweezing less painful. (And try not to be pre-menstrual, if at all possible.)

2 Get in front of a Truth Mirror. Not your lovely, flattering, bedroom mirror, but one that gets a direct hit of natural light and shows every pore and every flaw.

3 Tweeze away obvious stray hairs. If you want to be all fancy-like, hold a pencil vertically alongside your nose to the point where the pencil meets your eyebrow; this is the natural starting point for your brow. Tweeze the stray hairs between the two starting points, and from below your natural arch.

4 Do NOT tweeze above the brow and stay the hell away from that wax pot.

5 If you're a bit red afterwards, hold some ice over the inflammation, then cover up with some mineral makeup.

*Because you will have shaping appointments. On the scale of Beauty Rituals That Make a Big and Very Positive Difference to a Lady's Appearance, brows are higher up than blow-dries, manicures, facials and waxing.

# SOME GREAT AND HELPFUL EYEBROW TRICKERY AND TIPPERY.

**Oh, I do love this one:** Instead of buying an eyebrow brush, use a kid's toothbrush. Costs less; gives the same effect.

**This one's a cracker, too:** Clean up brows in between shaping sessions by framing them with highlighter. First, fill them in with your brow pencil/powder. Then, above and underneath the brow, draw a line of champagne-coloured highlighter, using a flat shadow brush and a creamy highlighter like the Multiple Stick in Copacabana from NARS, or Benefit's High Brow, a soft pink matte highlighter pencil intended for just this purpose. (Or, use concealer!)

**Can't forget this one:** I reckon a brow powder gives a more natural finish than a brow pencil – plus it's harder to stuff up. Buy a dedicated brow powder or, since eye shadows and brow powders are essentially the same, use an eye shadow the same shade as your eyebrows with an eyebrow brush.

**Or this one:** Filling in the brows is only half the job. You need to set your good work with either a dedicated brow wax or brow gel, such as MAC Brow Set.

(Investing in a brow palette with powders and waxes is a sound purchase; try Benefit Brow Zings or Clarins Perfect Eyes & Brows Palette.)

**And this one:** No brow gel? Pity. Use some hairspray on your index finger and groom into place.

**And, oh, this one too:** Condition brows regularly with castor oil.

**And this one:** Filling in gaps in your brows makes a huge difference to how they frame your face. Your easiest fix is a fortnightly tint, or you can fix any open spaces using short, irregular strokes of a brow pencil or brow brush to mimic the look of real hair (no heavy or thick lines). And follow the direction of the hair – if it goes straight up, so should your strokes. If it looks too harsh when you're done, soften it by wiping a cotton pad softly over the brows. (I tend to avoid the very beginning of my brows, as it can make them look too heavy.)

**Or this:** Blondes should go for blonde or taupe shades, auburn for redheads, and light brown or medium brown for brunettes.

# IF YOUR FRIEND WEARS TOO MUCH MAKEUP, SAY NOTHING.

How offensive! It's *her* face, yet you think you can just storm in with your feather boa (assumed) and cigar (probably) and snakeskin gloves (definitely) and tell her she is doing it all wrong? No, no, no.

'But!' you exclaim even though I can't hear you, 'I'm helping her look even MORE beautiful!' Well, that's subjective, unfortunately. But *okay*! Okay. Here are some techniques you can use. But remember to tread carefully, and also that, really, this is none of your goddamn business.

**Option 1:** Offer to do her makeup. This means you can do what you think will be flattering under the guise of a fun, girly getting-ready session. Be sure to tell her how gorgeous/wonderful/exciting her new look is.

**Option 2:** Ask her if she thinks YOUR look could do with a change. It probably can: makeup products and application should always be evolving, for all of us. Yes, you might learn how heavy-handed you are with blush, but it's fair and worth it, because then you will be given the chance to delicately suggest that you would love to see your friend without bronzer/hair extensions/so much lip liner one day.

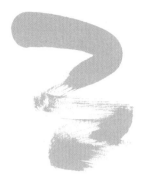

**Option 3:** Recommend an anti-product to one she uses too much of so you can coax her towards a new look under the guise of technical innovation. It might be some lovely, lightweight foundation, a less intense blush, or even a tinted version of the dark, dry, matte lipstick she wears. As with all of these tips, lead with positivity.

**Option 4:** Point out someone wearing simple, fresh makeup and tell her how great she'd look like that. If possible, choose someone who wears a lot of makeup, but who looks better when they lose 75% of it (like Johnny Depp). She may reveal why she wears a lot of makeup – whether it's habit, fear of not looking attractive or even unhappiness with her skin. This is *great*, cos it means you can really workshop some stuff, whether that's a different approach to her skin care, or an afternoon affirming her worth, power and gloriousness as a woman.

**Remember!** Your goal is not to criticise, but to illuminate potential new options, should they be of interest. Whether she takes on the advice is another thing altogether, because it's her face and her choice, and if she likes having very thin brows even though you can't stand them, it's her prerogative. I draw the line at greasy hair though. Wash that shit already.

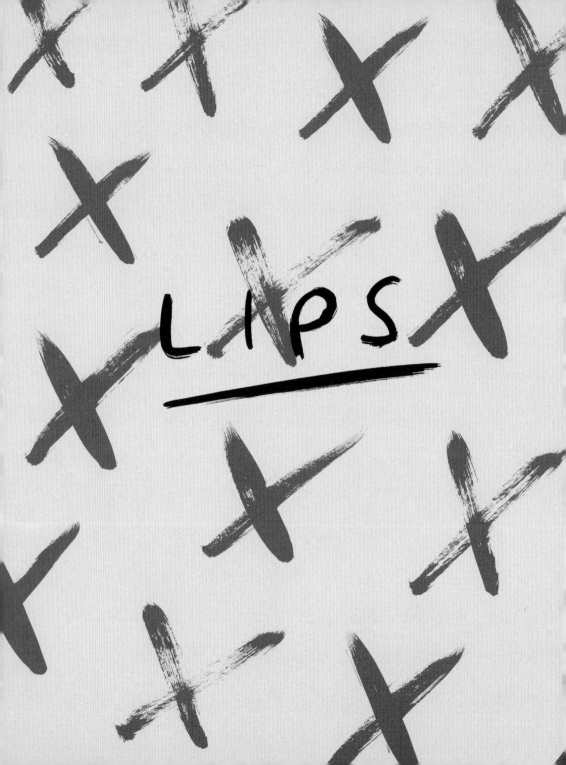

LIPS

Lip products are more fun than a sock full of frogs.

You can make people admire your chutzpah with bright neon-pink lipstick. Gasp at your elegance in a sheer berry stain. Force focus onto your heavily made-up eyes with a soft nude balm. Trick people into believing you time travelled from 1952 with a vibrant shade of crimson lipstick. Entice people to think about kissing you with a devastatingly juicy gloss. But you can also get cold sores. And dry flaky lips and stuff, too. Gross.

# HOW TO PROPERLY TEST A POTENTIAL LIPSTICK SHADE... AND THEN MAKE SURE IT WILL FLATTER YOU.

Chances are you're one of the estimated four frillion women whose lipstick looks different on their lips than when they sampled the shade on their wrist before purchasing it. This is because your wrist is about as similar in texture and colour to your lips as an orangutan is to an iPhone.

**Always test potential lip colours on the pad of your fingertip.** They are very similar in texture and colour and so it is a far more accurate testing ground.

SOME SHADES YOU'LL FIND PLEASINGLY FLATTERING:

**Fair skinned?** Go for soft browns that have a warm pink or peachy glow, or bold, exciting reds with a bluish tint. (Try Maybelline Color Sensational Lipcolour in Are You Red-Dy.)

**Olive skinned?** Nudes and light browns with warm tones, or brick-reds. Pops of colour like fuchsia and coral. (Try NARS Satin Lipstick in Honolulu Honey.)

**Dark skinned?** Deep reds with blue or purple tones, or deep reddish-browns. (Try Lancôme L'Absolu Rouge in Jezebel.)

*Hey! Try this!*

Blend foundation over the edges of your lips before applying lipstick: It makes the final shade look much more true to the colour of the actual lipstick.

*Or this!*

For a lazy, modern lipstick effect, use the tip of your middle finger to apply lipstick. The heat and oils from your fingertip melt the lipstick into your lips for a deliciously alluring stained effect.

# FIVE
## ways to un-dreary your face In winter.

### 1.

**Quench your miserable, thirsty skin.** Switch to a mousse, cream or oil cleanser, and use a hydrating face oil and/or serum underneath your moisturiser. And definitely exfoliate 2–3 times a week.

### 2.

**Fake vitality with vibrancy.** Bold, punchy lips teamed with healthy cheeks and defined, filled-in eyebrows do wonderful things for your face, teeth, eyes and mood. (So too does some gradual tanner.) My go-to is red-based orange lip, with a wash of soft bronze-copper on the eyes.

### 3.

**Brighten your head.** I call bullshit on that rule about summer being the best time to lighten your hair. Do it in winter when you NEED some light, I say! A few subtle, well-placed highlights around the face can do exciting things for your skin tone, eyes, makeup needs and probably even your reputation.

### 4.

**Piss that powder off.** Despite what the Department of Powder will tell you, the combination of dry skin and heavy, cakey, powder foundations isn't super cute. So, why not try switching to liquid or cream foundation? If you're scared because you have oily skin, try a liquid mineral, which usually has a semi-matte 'skin' finish and lasts ages, then set with loose powder.

### 5.

**Give yourself something fun to look at.** Paint your nails a fruity colour because bright, fun nail polish is statistically proven to lift your mood and ability to attract compliments, according to a study I just made up. So crack out the red, the orange, the melon, the coral, the burgundy – all the colours. This is no time for safe nudes, safeypants.

# REALLY BRIGHT LIPS ARE HERE TO STAY.

A punchy lip, be it orange or bright magenta or musky pink, is not to be thrown into the frivolous makeup basket anymore because bright lips are now a Classic Makeup look. Just as much as a smoky eye or an old Hollywood red lip. Oh, sure, yeah, I mean they started off all trailblazey and wild and, 'Holyshit, is...is that... are you...you can't be...is that *orange lipstick you're wearing*?!' a few years back, but we've come to accept that a bold pop of colour on the lips is just as relevant and chic and gorgeous as the aforementioned Iconic Beauty Looks.

**In my opinion a bright lipstick is best worn in a matte or creamy formula with:**

• Foundation and a dusting of powder on the eyelids to cover veins and create a flawless look

• Concealer to even out dark circles and cover blemishes and redness

• Mascara

• Blush

• Groomed brows.

But what would I know? Apart from everything.

*Bonus trick!*
*Vase-genius! Smear Vaseline along your teeth before applying bright lipstick to prevent said lipstick getting on your teeth. Or, mix it with lipstick for a dewy cheek sheen. Or, rub it around the neck of your nail-polish bottle to prevent the lid from sticking.*

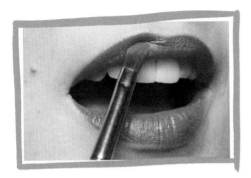

**Fun tip:** Apply bold lip colour right after your foundation to instantly energise your face and help you evaluate how much cheek and eye makeup you need.

**The small print:** A good complexion is kind of important when you're doing this look. This doesn't mean you need to have perfect skin, but you definitely need to create the illusion thereof with your foundation and concealer, because SO much focus is on the skin when:

a) The eyes are bare and,

b) While the focus is certainly on the lips, they will also strangely draw attention to the area surrounding them, kind of like a big spider on a white wall – you definitely notice how white the walls are when there is a whopping great spider on there. Spider chat! Sexy.

**I like...** Napoleon Perdis Dévine Goddess Lipstick in Hara for a bright orangey-red, MAC Vegas Volt for a true orange, Laura Mercier Lip Color in Tangerine for a coral-melon-pink, Revlon ColorBurst Balm Stain in Lovesick for a purpley-pink fuchsia, L'Oréal Color Riche Anti-Aging Serum lipstick in Freshly Candy for a musk pink, while NARS Funny Face is a fuchsia-berry pink that suits *all* skin tones.

# SOME HELPFUL TIPS FOR THOSE WHO ENJOY NATURAL, NUDE, MODERN LIPS.

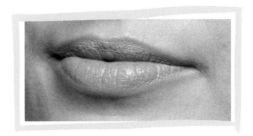

- For super massively natural lips, smudge a lip liner very similar to your natural lip colour into lips with your fingertip so there is zero sign of it, and yet it is definitely there somehow. Spooky. (Try Clinique Quickliner for Lips in Baby Buff.)

- Line and fill in your lips with a nude shade of stay-put liquid lipstick instead of lip liner – this removes the chance of Rank Outline Syndrome after eating/a few hours' wear and also makes lipstick last a *looot* longer. (Try: NYX Soft Matte Lip Cream in Buenos Aires or Athens.)

- Burt's Bees Tinted Balm in Hibiscus is a soft rosy-pink and is universally flattering. It gives lips a sleek, soft finish.

- Heavy, theatrical eyes demand an anti-lip colour to keep the face balanced. (Try MAC lipstick in Myth. Or don't. Up to you.)

- Morph a really vibrant cream blush into a subtle pastel lip colour by dabbing onto lips, then blending a nude lip or eyeliner pencil over it.

# GUMMY BARE AND FIND YOUR PERFECT NUDE GLOSS.

*Bonus trick!*
*Generally speaking, keep your lip gloss in the middle of your lips. Too much in the corners makes it look like you're drooling.*

**A given:** It's hard to find that Perfect Nude gloss. You know the one, it's a nudey beigey pinky latte shade that accentuates your lips' natural colour without overshadowing it, or stealing any of the focus from that incredible eye makeup you've done. It's not clear, and it's not opaque, it's just sheer and perfectly complementary to your lips, and face and makeup. It's the Holy Grail of lip gloss.

**A not given (a taken?):** Next time you're hunting for nude gloss, peel back your lips and look at the colour of your gums: a gloss that matches the exact colour of your gums will be the most flattering shade of 'nude' for your lips. Yes, you can hold up tubes of gloss to your gums in a department store. You *can*! Oh, come on. If anyone asks what you're doing you can share your new makeup tip and then you won't feel odd, because The Question Asker will be so grateful for your wisdom, she may even wish to hug you. (Probably don't allow it. You don't know where she's been.)

**Another given:** Jennifer Lopez clearly knew this trick a long time ago.

# RULES FOR LIPS THAT ARE RED.

I wore an outrageous, terrifyingly chic Red Lip recently (Tom Ford Lip Color Matte in Flame) and was quickly forced to recall Rules for Lips That are Red. And I thought, golly, am I glad I know what to do here or I could be in *real trouble*...

1 If you own a lip liner, now is when you would carefully fill in and outline the lips in a shade similar to the red you are wearing, or even a nude shade. If you are without liner, pat some concealer on your lips. (Make sure your lips are nice and moisturised first or you will get flakius maximus.)

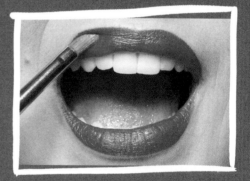

2 Use a lip brush (not the lipstick, you dingus!) to apply the lipstick. The stick itself is for out-and-about touch-ups only. Brush will give you precision and long lastiness. Especially on the corners.

3 Lightly top your lovely red lips with a coat of translucent powder (or blot with a tissue if you don't have any powder). Do the paint-powder 2–3 times in a row and your lip colour WILL NOT MOVE.

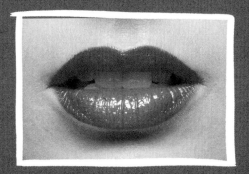

**4** Stick your index finger in your gob, and slowly remove. See how it takes excess lipstick! See how your teeth are saved from lipstick smears!

**5** Take a mirror out with you, and check your teeth and lips constantly. Red lipstick is attracted to teeth like nerds to an Apple store.

**6** There actually is no point six. Sorry. But there is a *compliment* six: 'Your lips look completely perfect.'

**A few red-commendations (hahaha!):** I like MAC Lipstick in Ruby Woo and Chanel Rouge Allure Luminous Intense Lip Colour in Pirate. For a softer finish, try a glossy stain, like YSL Rouge Pur Couture Glossy Stain in 11, Rouge Gouache, or a matte, lo-fi tint, like tarte LipSurgence Matte Lip Tint in Fiery.

Gloss fiend? Try Lancôme Juicy Tubes Lip Gloss in Cherry Burst over lips that are fully lip-lined in red.

*Bonus trick!*

*Try this vintage lip trick and enjoy the admiration of friends and strangers alike: First apply concealer around the lip line and stain lips with two shades of rich red. Use a dark red on the middle of the lips, and a medium red on the outside.*

# YOU CAN TOTALLY WEAR A DARK LIPSTICK. ALL OF YOU.

*Trick #1.*
*Light in the centre, whether it's a clear gloss or a hint of pink or red, will give dark lip colours warmth. So, if you've done a dark plum lipstick, a splodge of berry-toned gloss in the middle of the top lip will break it up.*

Wine- or plum-coloured lips were meant to remain locked in 1993. Everyone seems quite happy with that. But I'm not. Even the most chic and modern among us can wear vampish dark lips provided we leave our eyelids the hell alone.

You can go sheer, shiny or matte – up to you. (A berry-tinted lip stain is a nice, gentle way in.) But whichever way you go, please prep the lips with a nude/matching liner first and apply your product with a lip brush. You have about the same amount of room for error as a tightrope walker balancing above hungry velociraptors with such a dark colour, so be very precise and keep a mirror at hand for check-ups. If the colour is too intense, blot until it looks more stain-like.

*Trick #2.*
*Stop naughty lipstick from seeping outside of the lip line by tracing a cotton bud dipped in translucent powder around your lips before and after applying the lippie. No powder? Just use concealer or liquid foundation.*

Nicely mascara-laden lashes are a must, and some gentle bronzer will add warmth. Skipping the bronzer and sticking to just blush on the apples will keep things a little more elegant and vintage-looking, while a drawn-on moustache will confuse people into thinking you're a dapper French man.

*Trick #3.*
*Bronzed faces don't always demand a nude or a bright lip. Try a wine or burgundy lip stain or gloss instead. Daring! Exciting! Risky!*

**Products:** NARS Velvet Matte Lip Pencil in Train Bleu, MAC Mineralize Rich Lipstick in Lush Life, Revlon Super Lustrous Creme Lipstick in Black Cherry.

# WILL APPLYING GLOSS OVER AN INTENSE SHADE OF LIPSTICK SUCK? DEPENDS.

**Bonus trick!** Whenever you apply a very bright lip gloss, dab on some waxy concealer around the lips to soften the edges. (A stick concealer, ideally.)

**If you do add gloss all over lipsticked lips,** I hope you're unemployed, because you just landed a Full Time Job. Red, pink, orange and plum lips are hard work as is, but adding shiny, wet, slippery goo on top? Real difficult. A sloppy dribble of tinted gloss will be on your pegs and sneaking down to your chin before you can say, 'It appears I am a fool for doing this.'

**If you don't add gloss to lipsticked lips,** your lipstick will stay perfect and you can enjoy drinks and kisses and fettucine marinara without so much as a thought to your lips. Ha ha ha! As IF. If you've gone for a full, rich lipstick you've still locked yourself into an all-night contract with a mirror. Don't, and you risk That Disgusting Outline of Lipstick look. And that's enough to lose you friends.

**If you add just a dab of gloss in the centre of the lips,** you will add a very alluring pop of freshness and luminosity to what might have otherwise been a very serious lip situation. It will require a little more maintenance than if you were just wearing lipstick, but not nearly as much as if you applied the gloss all over.

# LOOK YOUNGER JUST BY CHANGING YOUR LIPSTICK.

**Buy creamy, hydrating lipsticks.** Or a dedicated anti-ageing one, like Clarins Rouge Eclat Lipstick.

Once we ladies hit A Certain Age, we need to start getting extra crafty with lipstick choices. So. Got some glue, cardboard and pipe-cleaners? *Good.* Now put them aside and focus for God's sake.

First of all, **chuck any shade of brown lipstick** that is darker than a latte. Ditto shades of **plum, wine and blood red**. Despite my advocating it on page 152, dark lipstick makes your lips look smaller and emphasises dark circles under the eyes. You can live without that. It also means you're at risk of being cast as the nasty school ma'am in movies.

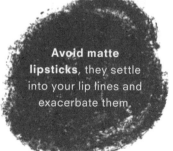

**Avoid matte lipsticks**, they settle into your lip lines and exacerbate them.

**Wear a gloss/lipstick hybrid** – the shimmer and gloss will make your lips look juicier and the lipstick will give good depth of colour. **Try:** Lancôme Color Fever Gloss or Estée Lauder Pure Color Gloss.

**A pink lipstick** a shade or two lighter than your natural lip colour will be intensely flattering and make you look years, decades, millennia younger.

**Consider a soft coral-based lipstick** – they're frightfully youthful and skin-brightening. **Try:** Bobbi Brown Rich Lip Color in Soft Coral, Rimmel Apocalips Lip Lacquer in Luna.

**Kick the lipstick all together** and wear a lip-plumping lip gloss. First fill in your lips with a nude-coloured lip liner, then apply a soft pink – no sparkle, please – lip gloss all over. A product with a built-in wand or applicator is better (for application and duration) than a tube that demands a sloppy finger-based application. (Also, see page 156 for a plethora of ways to make lips look fuller and more scrumptious sans collagen injections.)

# I'M GONNA GIVE YOU A FAT LIP.

According to Dr Larry Lipsfat,* plump, full lips are a sign of vitality and youth, which is why when we feel those things slip from our shiny red talons, we (often subconsciously) try to re-create the pillowy pout of a 16-year-old. Which I encourage (within reason).

**HERE ARE SOME WAYS TO DO JUST THAT:**

**Buy a lip-plumping gloss.** These give magnificent instant results. Sure, you might feel like you've rubbed your lips with pepper spray, but *leaping lip injectors* it's worth it. Try Fusion Beauty XL Advanced Lip Plumping Therapy, DuWop Lip Venom.

*Bonus trick!*
Put a smoodge of clear gloss in the indentation in the centre of your upper lip and in the centre of your lower one; it will make both look plumper.

*This person does not exist.

156

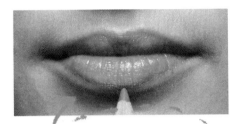

**The mini-liner trick.**
Draw a tiny line of 'nude' lip liner along the middle of your bottom lip. Apply your favourite lip colour all over as always. See how that slight line gives the illusion of a shadow, and fuller lips? Cool, huh.

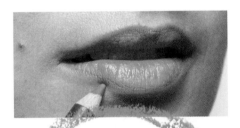

**Let someone inject you with collagen.** I'm yet to see a convincing, natural set of collagen-injected lips, but I *have* seen plenty of terrible, lopsided, lumpy, wongly, unattractive ones. Up to you, sweetlips.

**Outline your whole gob.**
Gently outline your lips with a neutral lip liner (try MAC Lip Pencil in Spice); start at the outer corner and follow the lips right around, making them just that little more oval than sharp on the edges. Then fill in your lips using a lip brush and your lipstick of choice.

**Let a friend bop you in the mouth.** A less popular option for obvious reasons (friends are hard to come by), but deeply effective in instantly fattening up the lips.

# ENJOY CHIC MATTE LIPS THAT AREN'T AS DRY AS OLD CRACKERS.

Matte lips are extremely elegant. They look and feel more grown up than shiny, glossy lips, and are for the woman who cares little for constant upkeep or annoying people who ask her the time when she is drinking her macchiato and reading *Financial Review*.

Problem is matte lipsticks, which are created to produce a lovely, dry finish, tend to use waxes rather than oils in order to make the lips less shiny, and these naughty waxes thieve moisture from your lips.

**So:**

• Make your dreamy, creamy hydrating lipstick LOOK matte, but not dry out your lips like matte lipstick do by using concealer as a base, then continuously layering on your lipstick, then tissuing off the excess until it looks suitably matte. Or just dust a bit of powder over your lipstick to tone down the shine.

• Or, use a matte lipstick but prime the lips first with a lip priming cream. These act like skin care (rather than a barrier, which can disrupt the look of your lipstick) and hydrate and fill in lines for a smooth appearance. Something like Too Faced Lip Insurance Lip Primer is great.

• Or just suck it up and use a matte lipstick, then gently exfoliate your lips with a warm washcloth and layer on a lovely lip serum or balm at night.

*Bonus trick!*

*Before taking a sip from a glass, discreetly kittylick it so your lipstick doesn't stick to the rim of the glass. God that looks disgusting.*

# UH, YOUR LIPS AGE TOO, YOU KNOW.

So why aren't you looking after them as you do the rest of your face and skin? For the love of lip liners, *get on board!*

**SPF:** Cover your lips in a broad-spectrum UVA/UVB balm when outdoors, or at the least, lipstick or gloss with SPF. And don't wear gloss to the beach – the shine just attracts the sun and will result in burned lips, pigmentation and even cold sores.

**Treat your lips:** In the same way your cute face needs nourishing, restorative face creams, masks and serums, so too do your lips. Using a good quality lip balm definitely helps, but a specialised treatment product with antioxidants and peptides will work a lot harder, and do more long term. One option is SkinCeuticals Antioxidant Lip Repair Restorative Treatment.

**Undo the damage:** If you have deep lip wrinkles from age, sun damage, disapproving lip pursing or smoking, Fraxel laser is a one-off, very effective treatment with only a few days' downtime. This is a single treatment and takes only a few days to heal. (But could never be accused of being cheap in a court of law.) (Also: cold sore alert – take lysine in the days leading up and have some Famvir tablets at the ready just in case!)

# LIP BALMS FEEL INCREDIBLY USELESS A LOT OF THE TIME.

I've had access to roughly 789 billion lip balms in my job, but so many left my lips dry after using them. No matter the price or the prestige, they leave my lips unhappy. Dry. Flaky. Irritated. Kickin' tyres and punchin' walls. But a lot of that comes down to me using them for the wrong thing. Because while all lip balms appear to vaguely have the same purpose – moisturise your lips – they do not. Most are actually lip barriers.

Lip barriers act as a protective layer to maintain whatever moisture you already have in your lips, but don't add any more. Where we lip balm lovers often come unstuck is using barriers for lip hydration, and then becoming annoyed when they give none. Petroleum (found in Vaseline and many popular pawpaw ointments) is a key example of this. And this is why you develop a reliance on these products: you're not actually getting any moisture for your lips when you apply, just a shiny wall on top of them, so you keep applying hoping for that nourishment. In addition, lots of lip balms have ingredients that topically feel nice but can cause dryness

and irritation (like eucalyptus, menthol and camphor).

The most effective lip product will have an occlusive barrier that seals in moisture, while simultaneously providing hydration with nice things like shea butter and sweet almond oil and jojoba.

**THE KEY TO AUTHENTICALLY MOISTURISED LIPS IS THREE-FOLD.**

**1** Exfoliate lips weekly. This removes the build up from balms, glosses and lipsticks and allows the next product to penetrate properly. Do this using a warm face cloth (or a dedicated lip scrub). Don't use a face scrub; too strong.

**2** Next, use a lip nourishing product (choose one with ingredients like vitamin E, sweet almond, coconut oil or shea butter) that contains no petroleum to properly rejuvenate the lips.

**3** Apply a lip barrier product to lock in that new lease of moisture. Use a lanolin-based product, ideally.

## A bonus trick!

Press some rosy pink eye shadow on top of plain lip balm for all-day colour. Delightful!

## One more:

Pawpaw contains the enzyme papain which is an exfoliant, so be mindful when you apply pawpaw ointment to your lips that you are gently removing dead skin cells – which is fine, except you should follow up with a hydrating lip product to replenish the lips. These ointments are fantastic for soothing bites, rashes, cuticles, dry heels, etc., but not lips, in my opinion. Also, some of them contain over 95% petroleum jelly, so read the dang label.

## Dear God, it's another one!

For DEVASTATINGLY chapped lips, do this once a day for a couple of days: swipe some honey onto your lips (being a humectant it cleverly draws moisture to the lips). After a few seconds apply a petroleum-free pawpaw ointment over the honey. Leave for 10–15 minutes then remove with a wet, warm cotton pad or face cloth. Apply a nourishing lip balm as normal.

PLUG!

*It would be remiss of me at this stage not to mention that since originally publishing this book, I have created my own 'perfect lip balm' after having been disenchanted with what was on offer. Even with the balms I did love, there was something…missing. They'd have a great feel or key ingredient, but then they'd ruin it with petroleum or camphor or eau de bubblegum. It's called Go-To Lips! and it incorporates all the lip superstars: ultra medical grade lanolin, shea butter, beeswax, vitamin E for antioxidants and eight sassy oils (sweet almond, apricot kernel, evening primrose, calendula, pomegranate seed, avocado, jojoba) to make sure the lips are nourished, but also have barrier protection, so you get to be lazier AND more hydrated.

# KILL OFF A COLD SORE IN 48 HOURS.

If there's one thing everyone loves, it's a cold sore. Both alluring and visually striking, they are the perfect way to jazz up a boring lip and the easiest way to guarantee a goodnight kiss from that dreamboat you've been eyeing off all night!

YEAH, RIGHT. Cold sores – hereafter CSs – are disGUSting. And I'd know, because I get them. Along with two-thirds of the population. But I have a technique that destroys CSs within 3–4 days, and not even my husband can tell I ever had one.

### Warning:
*If you don't get CSs, stop reading now, because this topic is revolting enough without non-sufferers turning up their noses and exposing nose hair at it in disgust.*

**THINGS YOU SHOULD ALWAYS HAVE ON HAND:**

- **Famvir or similar**\* (an oral famciclovir cold sore treatment you buy from the chemist). Not for the pregnant or breastfeeding.

- **Lysine** (an essential amino acid that fights the virus internally. Take one daily if you're prone to breakouts, and two twice a day during a breakout).

- **Acetone nail-polish remover and cotton pads/tips** (I buy the pre-made nail-polish remover pads for travel).

- **A sterilised pin/needle.**

- **Compeed cold sore patches** (keep a few in your wallet in case of sudden attacks).

**THINGS NOT TO DO:**

- Drink coffee

- Eat seeds, chocolate or tomatoes

- Stress out – it makes the little bastards worse

- Kiss people (unless you hate them)

162

### WHEN THE AREA IS HOT AND TINGLY, MOVE FAST

It can come down to minutes between a cold sore that lasts three days, and one that lasts 10. Immediately place a Compeed patch onto the site at the itchy stage: these are transparent hydrocolloid plasters that extract moisture from the sore and heal it, reduce pain, prevent spreading and keep things hygienic. Y'see, they treat the cold sore like a WOUND, whereas anti-viral creams try to suppress the herpes simplex virus, which is optimistic in my opinion. I avoid topical creams entirely.

Now quickly take your Famvir tablets, which will greatly lessen the time the cold sore hangs around, *but only if you take them on the first day of the sore manifesting*. Also, take some lysine.

### NO PATCHES ON HAND?

Put some nasty, strong acetone nail polish remover on a cotton pad and press it on the CS for a good, painful 15 seconds. Don't let any get into your mouth obviously, because it's toxic, and tastes rubbish besides. (Wash your hands once you're done.) This will dry the skin and remove the lovely, moist, bubbling, warm environment a cold sore needs to keep growing, and buy you enough time to get to the nearest chemist and buy some patches/Famvir.

Once you have your Compeed patches, use immediately. I often cut mine in half – having a weird, crinkled, plastic sticker on your face or lips isn't as cute as some might think. Use these from the blister stage, back-to-back, 24 hours a day, until the end of dry, flaky skin stage. (So, about two days longer than you think you need to.) They can prevent a scab occurring, they stop spreading and they minimise scarring. They are *wonderful*.

### WHEN YOU SEE BLISTERS, SORT THEM OUT

My (controversial) advice is to pop the blisters, otherwise they will keep growing and multiplying. Do it **carefully and hygienically**: wash your hands, then take a sterilised needle or pin, prick each blister separately, then very quickly blot with a small square of tissue to stop the serum weeping and spreading. Blot once, then toss straight in the loo. **If you don't take all hygienic precautions, you risk a new sore erupting**. Once the entire site is pricked and dry, 'sanitise' the area with acetone again. Place a fresh Compeed patch on straight away to stop spreading and reduce discomfort. Wash hands. You are in control, goddamnit!

**KEEP A PATCH ON AT ALL TIMES.**

Cold sores **do not need to breathe**. They need to suffocate and die. Keep liquids, foods and cosmetics, etc., away from the patch. At night or in the morning before work, wear your old one in the shower – **don't let the sore get wet!** – then remove once you're out. One patch will get you four hours through the day (food and drink weaken the adhesive), and all night. Before applying a new patch, hold some more nail polish remover on a cotton pad on the sore for 20 seconds to teach it who's boss.

**STAY VIGILANT**

By doing all of the above, my CSs go in 2–3 days. (In my teens they used to run well over two weeks, so this is a fucking miracle.) But! Just because you think it's gone, doesn't mean it is: CSs can rise again swiftly. So, keep on with the acetone/Compeed patches until there is NOTHING LEFT. Go past even the flaky dry skin bit.

**COVER-UP TRICKERY**

Now, during all of this, you might, annoyingly, have an event, and need to ditch the patches, as discreet as they are. Wear a patch till the last second, and put a new one on as soon as you're home.

**To cover a CS not on your lip:** Bravely just wear the patch because it makes the cold sore pretty invisible, or else remove it and buy a cheap lipstick brush (which you will toss post-CS) and delicately paint on a mix of foundation and creamy concealer – this will keep it dry and covered up. Avoid powder. It will need maintaining because your skin will flake. Sexy. One creamy, thick product I like for this (also brilliant for pimple hiding) is Shiseido's Sun Protection Stick Foundation.

**To cover a CS on your lip:** Use a thick, long-last, high-pigment liquid lipstick in a deep red. Two coats. It's opaque enough to cover the CS and keeps the area dry enough to help the healing carry on. Add bronzer and mascara, and no one, NO ONE, will know about your vile little lip terrorist.

I am arrogant enough to say that these tricks are definitely the best you'll ever read if you're a cold sore sufferer, and that they may change your life.

You're welcome.

*Many swear by Valtrex, which is way stronger than Famvir and will annihilate the CS much faster, but, at the time of publishing, Valtrex requires a prescription.*

3 out of 5 women won't mention cold sores or breakouts leading up to a big occasion because they know these things can sense fear, which they then use as a beacon to find the best location to set up their grotty little camp.

# IT'S TIME WE COMPLIMENT THE S OUT OF EACH OTHER.

I met a lovely sausage at an event recently who said knowing that she would be meeting me today, she put extra-special effort into her makeup.

But I barely heard her cos I was too busy criticising her blush and destroying her for wearing off-trend nail polish.

Kidding! Kidding. I kept the focus on her frizzy hair.

But seriously, I told her that her haircut was fresh and flattering, and her winged liner was a triumph, because it was, but also because I think we simply don't give enough compliments, and there is always room for more kindness in the world, and also peanut butter–based treats. I also assured her that it is the woman who writes beauty books claiming to be an expert who should be under scrutiny, *not* the delightful member of the public, and also for her to please not notice the big pimple on my chin.

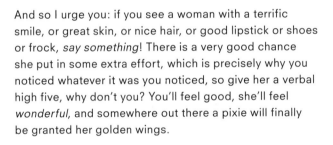

And so I urge you: if you see a woman with a terrific smile, or great skin, or nice hair, or good lipstick or shoes or frock, *say something*! There is a very good chance she put in some extra effort, which is precisely why you noticed whatever it was you noticed, so give her a verbal high five, why don't you? You'll feel good, she'll feel *wonderful*, and somewhere out there a pixie will finally be granted her golden wings.

**Extended remix:** if you really like a lady's hair or brows, or appreciate the glow of her skin, ask her where she goes/what she uses. Accumulating a solid, reliable, talented Beauty Army can be a long and frustrating process of trial and error (and shocking spray tans), especially if you have moved to a new state/country/planet, so work smart not hard by getting recommendations from women who are clearly and visually in the know, if their fluttery, perfect lash extensions are anything to go by.

# HAIR

There's simply nothing like a fresh haircut or exciting new colour or blow-dry or Excellent Hair Day to make you feel terrific and confident and sexy and attractive and polished and gorgeous!

(Except maybe a couple glasses of champagne.)

90% of women notice that
100% of men do not notice
when they change their hair,
but 100% of men say that
only 40% of women notice
when they change theirs, so
100% of men think that women
should ease up on them
by at least 50%.

# YOUR FACE SHAPE AND YOUR HAIRCUT NEED TO BE GOOD FRIENDS.

**HERE'S QUITE A FUN WAY TO FIND THAT FACE SHAPE:** Pull your hair off your forehead with one hand, look into a mirror and trace the outline of your face on the glass with lipstick. How mischievous! And yet so useful.

**IF THE OUTLINE IS BASICALLY A SQUARE:** You want your hair to have soft edges and layers, and you definitely don't want severe, angled bobs or very blunt fringes, which will amplify broad jawlines or strong chins.

**Cuts:** Whatever length you prefer, ask your cutter for graduated layers around the face, choppy ends and long, dreamy fringes.

**Styling:** Curls and waves are great for softening, especially with a centre part and some face-framing layers.

**IF THE OUTLINE IS BASICALLY A CIRCLE:** Your cheeks are hiding your cheekbones, so let's create the illusion of some with your hair. Probably don't go for a super short or mushroom (all the volume around the ears) style, as all that will do is point fingers to the roundness of your face.

**Cuts:** Longer hair with layers that frame the face, with some layers being cut to end at (and graze) the top of the cheeks, which creates the look of angled cheekbones. Short hair (if you can keep it longer than your chin, that would be a real bonus, as that makes the face look a little longer) with haphazard, choppy ends will add contrast and interest and angles.

**Styling:** Keep the layers close to your face and go for an off-centre-part to counter the roundness.

**IF THE OUTLINE IS BASICALLY AN OVAL:** You're in luck – you can pretty much do what you like. Because your face is equal parts soft and angular, you don't need to rely on balancing cuts or styles.

**Cuts:** How are you feeling today? Like you might enjoy a feisty crop? Do it! Like you might suit long, lusty layers? Do it! Like mimicking Lady Gaga's latest wig? *Go sick. The world is your hair salon.* If, however, your face is on the longer side, perhaps entertain a long, sweeping fringe, or cut in some layers that end at your chin.

**Styling:** The oval-faced can get away with pretty much any hairstyle, you lucky little lemur. (Again, if your face is a little longer, choose side-parts over centre-parts to offset the length.)

**IF THE OUTLINE IS BASICALLY A CHRISTMAS TREE:** You might be prematurely excited about December 25.

171

# FIVE
## *ways to fix a bad haircut.*

Bad chop, huh? You're not alone, girl. I know this because I'm looking into your home and can see other people around you. But also you are not alone in the shitty haircut stakes. Aside from snappy wigs, extensions and fedoras, here are some of your options:

## *1.*

**Embrace texture.** In my opinion ('fickle and unsubstantiated since 1980!'), hair rarely peaks when it is unstyled, flat and freshly washed. So get your styler or curling tong out and play around one night. It's amazing the difference some texture and waves can do to a cut. (And how well they disguise bad ones.)

## *2.*

**Try some new products.** If you've gone from simple, longish hair you knew exactly how to style to something alien and unpredictable, *go with it*, don't try to push it into What You Know. Shorter hair usually benefits from things like sea salt spray, wax, pomade and styling cream, as they give lift, texture and a modern look. Go for products that give subtle texture with a believable finish, nothing crunchy or sticky. (Examples are Bumble and bumble Texture Hair(un)dressing Créme, and Redken Powder Grip 03.)

*4.*

**Slick and styled.** Tucking slick hair behind the ears (or just one ear) is always chic, as is a low pony at the nape of the neck with a deep side part up front. Wet your hair and apply some gel (or even straightening balm) through it, then use a fine-tooth comb to neatly style it into place.

*3.*

**Accessories and trickery.** Try using bobby pins to secure little twists of hair pulled back off the face, backcombing a quiff up front, making a fake fringe by pulling hair from the front in a side part and tucking behind one ear, or just blow drying it smooth and popping it up into a bun, top knot or pony.

*5.*

**Go back.** Head back to the salon and tell them you really, really don't like your new hair, even after a few days of chatting to it over Chai lattes and trying to get to know it better. They want you to be happy – it's in their best interest, because bad publicity is, well, bad – so they will probably either try to fix it, or at least help you with styling.

But who knows? Sometimes we resist change for so long that the universe (or a distracted hairdresser) steps in to take care of it for us… It might just be the beginning of a Brand New You!

Or you will just wear it back every day until you're happy with it again.

# THE MOST FLATTERING HAIR COLOUR FOR YOUR SKIN TONE.

Look, you can have whatever the heck hair colour you want. Of course you can. But some, whether you like it or not, will be more flattering for your skin tone than others. Some will make your skin look fantastic and your eyes dazzle, and some will wash you out like a filthy old dishcloth. And if you get to the end of this sentence and start the next one, and then keep reading from there, you will learn which ones are which.

The first thing to do is work out if you're cool or warm-skin toned. So go to page 66 and work it out already.

**Warm?** Go for colours that can be described as gold, beige, sunkissed or honey. If you prefer darker hair, choose a warm, golden brown or auburn, coppery reds. The key, in case you missed all the hints, is to stay warm, and avoid colours with cool or ashy tones. And super massively avoid very extreme shades like ebony, white or violet. Unless you're in a band and the washed-out look is crucial to your image.

**Cool?** Just like the warm guys choosing warm colours, you should choose cooler tones to match your skin tone. Ash (even platinum) blondes can work (especially if you are naturally fair) as can cool, flat browns, and blue-based, cool, cherry or ruby reds. Probably give buttery, gold, yellow blonde tones or bronzey reds a miss.

Of course, a professional colour consultation is ALWAYS worth having, because while skin tone is helpful when determining which hair colour will make you look most magnificent, so too are things like eye colour and the kind of makeup and tan you sport.

Of course #2, there are always exceptions, and some people suit many different hair colours. Just ask Katy Perry. (I have her fax number if you need it.)

# ONE, TWO, HOW MANY TIMES DO WE SHAMPOO?

The kids in the salon always shampoo your mop twice because they know that the first wash is to clean the hair and the second wash is to treat the hair, as per whatever shampoo you use claims to do (colour protect, revitalise, banish frizz etc.).

Pause. Repeat.

**1st shampoo:** Clean.

**2nd shampoo:** Treat.

**OTHER SHAMPRULES:**

• If you wash every day cos your hair is very fine: **You may shampoo just the once**. (Also, consider skipping conditioner altogether.)

• Twice, three times a week washer? **Two quick shamps**.

• Use lots of silicone or hair dusts or powders or texturisers or heavy hair products? **Twice. Always twice**.

• And if you're only washing your hair once a week: **You better be shampooing that nest twice**. And thoroughly. *Dang.*

• Alternate route: **Use a clarifying shampoo**. They're designed to remove build-up. I like O&M Original Detox Deep Cleansing Shampoo.

*Bonus trick!*
*Don't spray hairspray directly onto your hair – spray it onto a paddle brush and then groom your hair with that. Prevents build up and stickiness.*

# WHEN YOU APPLY A HAIRSTYLING PRODUCT TO YOUR HAIR...

*Think.*

Whether that is a mousse, straightening balm, anti-frizz serum or dry shampoo, where do you apply it first?

Just think about it for a second.

Most of the time, we put it onto our hands, and then our hands go straight to the front and top of our head. Which is the precise place you DON'T want excess styling product, because the minute you have any grease or heaviness there, *your whole hair looks lank.*

So, in general (unless it's a root booster or lifter), keep your paws and your product away from your scalp, fringe and the front layers. Start at the mid-lengths instead and take the product down to the tips. (At the very least start at ear level.) When you comb the product through, you will automatically carry some back up to the root area, and that little amount is all you need. Really.

# YOU NEED TO OWN SOME MOUSSE.

It's the foundation of hair styling. The trick is to choose a modern-day mousse; key words to look for include body, flexible, lightweight and volume.

**How to apply mousse is simple:**

- Measure out a 4.5 × 8.2 mm portion of mousse and put aside in a Petri dish to set.

- Now, taking a titanium fine-tooth comb and a stainless-steel kebab skewer, transfer the mousse to the hair, taking care not to go any higher than 1.67 cm off the scalp.

- Apply heat from a blow-dryer to the moussed sections, but ONLY with the nozzle facing at a 49% angle and at a heat of 60°C.

**Alternatively, you could just do this:**

Spray mousse onto your hand, and run through the hair from the mid-lengths to the tips when your hair is damp and freshly washed, or dry and clean-ish. Then brush through thoroughly so the whole head has product. Now when you blow dry, you'll get volume, and even if you use a flat iron after blow drying, you will still have body and movement.

**Products:** L'Oréal Professional Tecni Art Volume Lift, John Frieda Luxurious Volume Bountiful Body Mousse.

# HOW TO LET CURLY/ FRIZZY/WAVY HAIR DRY (MOSTLY) NATURALLY, AND NOT HAVE IT LOOK LIKE SHIT.

When Proper Styling is as appealing as finding a large hair in one's pasta, but allowing your hair to dry by itself is out of the question (because it will be wild and bushy), you must use a product that will assist the transition from 'Wet and manageable hair' to 'Dry and sort of decent looking hair'. Here are some options:

### A STYLING CREAM

Run this through wet hair (avoiding the roots) and then comb it through. It tames frizz but also adds just that touch of weight you need for keeping curls looking like curls, and not like deranged, dry, brittle fairy floss.

**Try:** Bumble and bumble Curl Conscious Defining Creme, Davines LOVE Curl Cream.

### SOME HAIR DUST

If boofy, fluffy, too-clean hair is a problem, a sprinkle of this at the roots (tap onto your fingers and work through if you're a rookie) all over the scalp (on dry hair) will instantly give you sexy, textured, Second Day Hair.

**Try:** Aveda Pure Abundance Hair Potion.

### A THERMAL PROTECTANT SPRAY

Actually a product intended for protecting hair from the use of stylers and curling tongs. But while using it for this exact purpose (a purpose it serves very well, incidentally), I discovered that if applied to hair that is 80–90% dry, and combed through, it is pretty great for creating lovely, rounded curls, and saying 'beat it' to frizz. As in, I didn't even have to use my curling tongs in the end, because the curls suddenly behaved so nicely. And as a bonus, it smells like the kind of cocktail you can only order on holidays.

**It is:** evo Icon Welder Hot Tool Shaper.

## A SEA-SALT/BEACH-HEAD SPRAY

This stuff gives grit and texture; just spritz it through, all over (flip your head and do the underside too), and then allow it to dry. (If you're feeling cheaty, blast your hair with a hair dryer on high heat as this will give you even more texture and root lift too.) I highly recommend using sea-salt spray if you're going to create messy plaits and braids and so on, because your hair will have more grip and more texture.

**Try:** O&M Surf Bomb, Oribe Dry Texturizing Spray. (This is a gorgeous mutant of texturiser, dry shampoo and light hairspray; I love it for completely crunch-free texture that moves.)

*Bonus trick!*
*If your mirror is being all stupid and steamed up, blow your hair dryer on it, on high heat for 10 seconds, to clear the fog.*

# SO YOU WANT CURLS AND VOLUME?

There's no denying you're greedy, but I see your point: volume is crucial, both to keep the hair from dropping if you have straight or fine hair, and for longevity of style. You have a few options for big, bouncy, full, smooth curls that last (whether natural or artificial). Sadly, none of them involve eating pecan pie. Shame. Such a delicious pie.

**OPTION ONE:**

Use a thickening lotion throughout your hair before you style/create your curls. These are multi-purpose: they fatten up the hair, smooth it and (should usually) prevent your hair from heat-styling damage.

**Suggestions:** I like Redken Thickening Lotion 06 All Over Body Builder – but use only a tiny amount!

**OPTION TWO:**

Use a body-building mousse. This is a stylist's absolute favourite backstage product for the exact thing you're doing with your hair. *They all use mousse!* Mousse and hairspray. And coffee. (For their brains. Not the hair.) Try something with words like 'volume' or 'body' or 'thickening' in the title.

**Suggestions:** Kevin.Murphy BODY.BUILDER, PHYTO Professional Intense Volume Mousse.

**OPTION THREE:**

Use a root-lift spray at, uh, the roots, and then run a heat-protecting curl booster through the rest of the hair. Blow dry smooth all over then get to work creating fetching, glamorous brushed-out curls! Do this by creating curls all over the head with a curling tong (or hot rollers). Wait 10 minutes (because hair sets when it is STONE COLD! So let it get stone cold) then gently brush out your stiff curls with a cushion brush. Lightly mist all over with a light-hold hairspray. (For extra glamour, gently backcomb sections with your brush before smoothing over them.)

**Suggestions:** I like evo Liquid Rollers Curl Balm for this, or Goldwell StyleSign Twist Around.

**AND OH, DEFINITELY READ THIS BIT:**

Use day-old hair for creating curls. The curls will set and hold much better, and last longer. Clean hair is too slippery and ridiculous and the curls will fall out.

*Bonus trick!*

*Wrap – never clamp – your hair around the curling tong barrel for softer, more natural waves.*

88% of women believe their hair looks perfect the day before they are booked in to have it cut and coloured. Similarly, 74% of women attract the most compliments on their hair when it's at its filthiest. This makes 100% of them quite annoyed.

# ON THE TOPIC OF
# RAZORED HAIR CUTTING...

Razor cutting is done with a razor blade (who would have thought!), which means the hair is cut on an angle. Your stylist will glide the razor down the hair shaft, which makes it thinner and pointier at the ends, rather than the sharp line scissors give. It's excellent for making hair lighter (especially on men with sheep's wool hair) and can be a marvellous tool in the right hands and on the right hair. But it can also lead to a walloping great mess, especially if your stylist is new to the game, or you have curly hair, or you try doing it yourself with your Gillette Venus.

**Good for:** those with very thick or coarse hair, as it makes the hair lighter and gently softens the ends. It also works well for very straight (and moderately wavy) hair. Asian hair responds very well to razor cutting because it creates movement in very straight (mostly thick) hair. If you want a shaggy or wispy hairstyle or fringe (as opposed to a sharp one), razoring is terrific. Razor cuts also work on super-short pixie-style cuts and on edgy layered hair, and it will beautifully soften a very sharp bob and create a lovely angled, graduated line. (a.k.a. Gwyneth Paltrow with her old classic one-length, shoulder-skimming cut.)

**Less good for:** fine, limp, curly or frizzy hair. It will just amplify the problem. My hair is *all* these things, which is why when I had my hair razored, things didn't go so well. I had ends that looked like they'd, well, been attacked with a razor. And razor cutting is not meant to look like it was razored; it's just meant to give texture and to soften. If you want your fine hair to appear and feel thicker, maybe try a one-length, 'paintbrush ends' scissors cut, not a layered razor cut.

If you feel like you might be a good candidate for a chic angled bob, or a lovely wispy long cut, or just want to lose weight from a heavy, thick mop, razor the heck on. If you have very curly or frizz-prone hair, give it a wide berth.

# THE FINE HAIR WEIGHT-GAIN PROGRAM.

If there is one thing people with fine hair want to know, it's what a group of sharks is called. The answer, obviously, is a shiver. Another thing they often want to know is how to elegantly, subtly boost the amount of body and volume in their hair. Here are some ways:

**The cut.** A blunt bob can offer depth and texture with the right styling/products, layering around the face will add some movement and texture, and if you have straighter hair, a longish side fringe can do wonders for adding shape and excitement.

**Some colour.** Flat hair colour makes your hair look... flat. Go for some highlights or lowlights to create the illusion of depth. (Also, peroxide adds volume, *yassss!*)

**Wash with a shampoo for fine hair** and only apply conditioner from the mid-lengths to the ends. Or don't use traditional conditioner; instead mist a light leave-in conditioner through the lengths of towel-dried hair.

**Use root-lift product,** flip your head upside-down and apply all over your scalp before you style your hair. Makes a big difference. (Literally.)

**For modern, soft, 'big' hair** use a thickening spray or mousse all throughout dry hair, and blow dry through. Then use a small curling iron to create curls all over your head. Let the curls cool completely, then brush hair out and back comb or tease for even more volume. Lightly mist with a flexi-hold hairspray for hold. (See also page 180 for creating curls.)

**Feed your hair hamburgers.**

*Did you know...*

*Aeroplanes make your hair flat. Wash and style with a root-lifting/body-building/thickening product before you board, then pull up into a very high loose bun on your head once on board to keep the volume.*

# THE ONLY WAY TO GET YOUR HAIR ALARMINGLY STRAIGHT WITH STYLERS.

Is simple. And every hair stylist does it when they are straightening hair. *All of them*. And yet, even after seeing it roughly 563 times, we still don't do what they do when using our stylers at home.

**You must first comb the section of hair you're straightening.** Comb it with a styling comb or tailcomb, and then follow immediately after with your styler. The combing, obviously, gets rid of all knots and smoothes the hair, making life really easy and fun and enjoyable for the styler to glide through without a care in the world. The result is smooth, dead-straight hair and no naughty waves or curling up at the ends.

Of course, using a good thermal protectant before you style your mop helps your cause, too. Heaps. I like Tresemmé's, and also R+Co's One Prep Spray.

# YOU MIGHT WANT TO CHANGE THE WAY YOU BLOW DRY YOUR HAIR.

Sometimes I learn a hairstyling technique that makes my brain pause and get out its brain pen and brain notepad and write a little brain note. This was one of them.

It concerns blow drying your hair straight. And not destroying it in the process. You see, for years people like me have encouraged people like you to use a barrel brush (natural bristle or thermal) when blow drying your hair straight. Which still stands, but switching to a styling brush and wrap-drying your hair for the bulk of your actual *drying* (as opposed to *styling*) definitely does less damage.

**What's wrap-drying?** It's when you're drying your hair with a hair dryer, and you slowly run a styler (or 'Denman', which is a brand name, like Esky) brush through damp hair from root to tip, back to front, side to side, flipping the hair over to each side of the head and generally just really having a fun time taking your hair in every direction, almost as though you are gently creating hair turbans, or wrapping the hair over and around the head. You don't section the hair, you don't go over each section 567 times as you might with your barrel brush, you just gently dry the hair off all over, without any tangling or pulling or grabbing that barrel brushes can be prone to doing. (Be sure to flip that hair all over the head and dry it in every which-way for a thorough dry-off – with volume – that will last.)

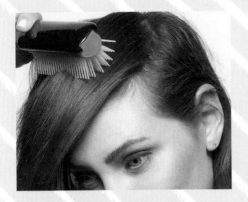

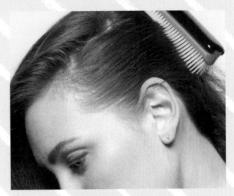

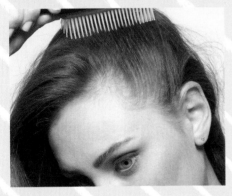

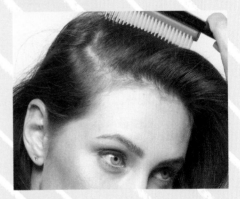

**Why it's called wrap-drying:** Back in The Day, before hair dryers and stuff, women would brush and then wrap the hair around the head before pinning it in places as it dried – which lengthened and straightened out curls and waves.

**Why it's better:** You do FAR less damage to the hair. And with the invention of ceramic styling irons, there really is no need to 'blow dry' the hair straight; instead, we can just dry it gently, without pulling and tugging excessively, then use a styler to get it smooth.

**Small print:** I still use my barrel brush sometimes, of course. Especially to straighten the naughty front sections and get rid of cowlicks. But the gentle wrap-drying followed with my irons looks just as good, gives loads of volume, is just as straight (straighter, even?) and I don't feel nearly so guilty making my hair straight. Of course, I always apply a thermal protectant before using ANY brush and heat combo. I'm no dingus.

# DO I NEED A 'SALON' HAIR DRYER? WHAT DOES THAT EVEN MEAN?

An emphatic YES! from the ZFB camp.

• They are much, much faster.

• They have the wattage needed for styling that works, and lasts.

• They are far less damaging: salon-grade hair dryers will generally have ionic, tourmaline or ceramic energy which cuts your blow drying time by about 889%. Plus, since the cuticle covering of the hair shaft doesn't get blasted open (and damaged – which is what shitty hair dryers do, and which causes frizziness and a ratty finish) and moisture is trapped in rather than 'boiled out', the hair is smoothed and nurtured as it's dried. Yew!

• They last FOR AGES. They're made for salon pros who use their hair dryer all-day, everyday, and are well-built with powerful motors.

I use a very lightweight, easy-to-handle, wonderfully long-corded Parlux 3200 Ceramic & Ionic Hair Dryer, which I have had for six years and counting. It looks like hell now, but is such a reliable, gorgeous, powerful son of a gun.

While a Parlux might cost a bit more – around $150, say – six years of Pretty Great Hair and not one issue is worth it. And anyway, how much did you spend on that styler again? Over $200? And yet you use your hair dryer just as much, if not more? Interesting.

All of that said: 'consumer' hair dryers have come a long way. Many have ceramic or ionic technology, and are fine if you have short hair, or you literally just 'dry off' and don't go over many times or straighten daily. But they do lack the horsepower of a pro-dryer, and *can* burn your hair with their crazy one-setting heats, or, if they have no fan cage, might even pull your dingin' hair into the motor! Imagine that. Or, if you're me, *remember* that, cos it happened.

**NO MATTER WHICH HAIR DRYER YOU CHOOSE,
HERE'S WHAT YOU WANT FROM IT:**

**Several heat settings.** I only use high heat for the initial 'dry-off' when the nozzle ISN'T attached, then switch to medium heat for styling and repeated going-over of the hair. For second-day refreshing and re-styling, low-heat, nozzle on, and the appropriate brush is the way to go.

**High and low power settings.** High for drying; low for styling.

**At least 1600 wattage.** Mine is 2000, which is salon-strength and EFFING FANTASTIC.

**A long nose.** This allows you to really get in there and direct heat where you need it, especially at the back of the head.

**A slanted nozzle for precise styling, and a diffuser.** Diffusers are underrated and very excellent for scrunching and drying curly hair into non-fluffy curls (use high heat, low power).

**A cool-shot button.** Hair sets when it's STONE COLD (the cold air closes off the cuticle) so always blast your finished, blow-dried hair with cold air for a minute at the end to set it.

**Ionic, tourmaline or ceramic technology.** Faster, less damaging, traps moisture in the hair, reduces static electricity, etc., etc., etc.

**Can make a fantastic martini.** Crucial for obvious, pretendy reasons.

# THE FASTEST WAY TO BLOW DRY YOUR HAIR YOU NEVER KNEW...

Will be with a vented barrel brush that has the words **tourmaline, ceramic, ionic or thermal** in its name (see page 257 if you want to know what the brush looks like).

Don't use them on wet hair, though. Use a Tangle Teezer or a Denman (see page 163) on wet hair, because they don't tug and tear and damage. Use a vented barrel brush once your hair is about 50% dry, to smooth it, straighten it, curl it and shape it, and marvel at just how rapidly it does these things.

**Fun fact! A larger barrel will give you more volume; a smaller one more precision (good for fringes).** There. See? You've read one little paragraph and you've already got something to tell the girls at After Work Drinks on Friday, just as soon as Jemma has finished telling that story about when she got home from personal training and was totally counting on eating that left-over Thai for dinner, and then she discovered her flatmate had EATEN it. I mean, who DOES that?

*Bonus trick!*
*To make your blow dry last a few days, don't finish with a serum or hairspray. (If you're in the salon don't let them do it.) Instead, use a lightweight mousse before you blow dry. Much better.*

# YOU ARE COMPLETELY DESTROYING YOUR HAIR, YOU KNOW.

If you have lovely, natural hair that dries perfectly, then you don't need to read this.

Okay, now that *she's* gone, let's discuss how you can stop ruining your hair so much provided you heat style as much as I do.

### HEAT STYLING:

Using tools like hair dryers, curling irons, stylers/straighteners and even thermal/ceramic/tourmaline brushes.

### WAYS TO MINIMISE DAMAGE:

**Use a weekly mask or treatment and have a cut every 6–8 weeks.** Blasting hot air onto your hair opens the cuticle layers of the hair. This is no good. Conditioners and treatments will definitely help, but too much blow drying (plus lots of colouring etc.) will result in a Massive Beauty Product Fail, because once the cuticle layer is shot, the hair is all weak and shit and breaks off and all you can do is SNIP.

**Beware the nozzle.** Blow drying your hair with that little nozzle on the end *is as bad as using a styler or tongs* because it is such a concentrated hit of intense heat. So if you're just 'drying' not actually 'styling' your hair, drop the noz. (Go down a brush size if you need more precision in your styling.)

**Protect every time.** When you use straighteners and tongs, you are placing a 220-degree implement tool on your hair. For many minutes at a time. Sizzle! Scorch! Burn! You must ALWAYS prep the hair first with a thermal protectant product (see page 161). Either apply on towel-dried hair before drying, or on dry hair, mist it in section by section as you tame, straighten or curl.

**Wear a novelty Santa hat.** This not only looks stylish and eliminates the need for all heat styling, but is a particularly good conversation-starter when worn in August.

# (THE FUTILITY OF) BATTLING FRIZZ WHEN HUMIDITY IS AT 498%.

If you think you can have great hair on a humid day, no offense, but you are a goose. You must let the dream of straight or flawless hair go for the day and utilise the specific trickery and artillery humidity demands.

## PREP

**Frizz-fighting/smoothing shampoo and conditioner.** Any clever stylist hair person type will tell you that prevention starts in the shower. Coat your hair with mild smoothing agents as you wash and it *will* make a difference to your styling.

**DEFINITELY use an anti-frizz serum.** A pea-sized amount in dripping wet hair. That's the way to use it. (You can also apply on frizzy ends when hair is dry.) Ol' mate Johnny Frieda does an extra strong version, which is ideal when you're in battle. I wouldn't blow dry too much – it tends to make the hair even more ridiculous and lank and unmanageable once you step outside. Also, it is futile. Just do the fringe if you must.

**Use a smoothing or taming styling product from the mid-lengths to the ends only.** This could be your blow-dry cream, a leave-in conditioner, a styling cream, a frizz serum – anything that will add some weight. Also, a root-lifter is a surprise winner – volume is a good thing to have at the roots when you're dealing with frizz.

**Don't forget the Old School stylers.** Gel and hairspray are exceptional at fighting frizz and keeping hair in place, and I strongly suggest you buy and use both. And a tailcomb for creating slick, deep side-parts and neat low buns (see page 198). So elegant with some lovely large earrings or a scarf, or a pet parrot perched on your shoulder.

*Bonus trick!*
*Use hand cream or*
*coconut oil to smooth your*
*hair down if you're, like,*
*really desperate.*

## STYLING

**Daytime:** Your best and most chic option is a low bun/pony or an adorable top knot. Work with dirty hair by spraying in a little dry shampoo or volume dust and scruffing it up. Or, pins! Use lots of bobby pins and clip back little sections of fringe or front bits (if your hair is short, just clip back the fringe to one side and show everyone how ambivalent you are about the humidity) and embrace el relaxo wild hair.

Centre-parts are a JOKE in humidity, so maybe flip the part over to one side, along with a fair chunk of your hair, and be all Jerry Hall. Scrunch through a little bit of hair oil and comb it back into a low pony or bun. Or, do a low side plait, or work in a cool braid across your forehead. You know, cool things.

**Night-time:** Put it back. Seriously, don't waste time styling or blow drying. And try not to wash your hair, if possible. Fluff and frizz make a spectacularly powerful combo. If your hair is looking a bit rubbish, wet it and slick it back. Work in some styling cream or gel and comb it through then tie at the nape. If your hair is dry and looking textured and decent, leave it be (and crack out some eyeliner), or do a sexy half-up, half-down, or pull it round to one side and do a messy side-bun/plait. Remember: The idea is not to fight the frizz, but work with it. Or completely slick it down into submission like you are some kind of sicko hair dominatrix.

**Or:** Surrender. Go feral. Go big. Go wild. Suck it up. *Rizz the Frizz!*

# FIVE

## bad hair day fixes.

Unlike the cheerful, singing women portrayed in Disney movies, our hair is not always thick, luscious and alluring. Which is annoying, but we get on with life. Unless we're premenstrual and hungry and running late, in which case it's The End Of The World.

Here are some common hair issues, and the fixes I use with heedless abandon. This is a sight to behold, because a woman without heed is a terrifying thing indeed.

### 1.

**Your roots (really) need doing.** It depends where your roots are. My highlights are applied in a side part, so for me to flip my part to the other side (my usual advice for root-disguising) or do a centre part, or even a fully slicked back look, is actually worse. So, I spray in dry shampoo, which masks the darkness and fluffs it up a bit. If it's *real* bad, I mist sea salt spray all over while my head is flipped upside down, then blast it with the hair dryer on high for 30 seconds. This musses it all up, making me look cooler than I am, and like the roots are 'intentional'. Pulling it up into a top knot is usually the best move from here.

### 2.

**You need your hair to look 'fancy' in 120 seconds.** Grab a fistful of mousse and mash it through dry hair, then smooth with a hair dryer on high heat. Take your curling tong or styler and do about 10 big curls all over the head, randomly and furiously. Pay little heed to where. WE ARE HEEDLESS WOMEN, REMEMBER. Spray lightly with hairspray and leave crunchy to set. Do your makeup as they cool for five minutes. Now, comb your fingers through the curls. Shake them out and marvel at the instant volume and body. Finally, scrape back your hair loosely and tie into a loose pony at the nape of your neck. Take the 'pony' bit and bobby-pin pieces of it into a fancy bun-chignon thing. The wispier and more bulbous, the better. Gently wisp and tug a few micro-pieces out around your face too. Add interesting earrings or a neckpiece to jazz up. Well. Look at *you*, jazzy!

## 4.

**You have too-dirty hair that just does THE WRONG THING no matter what you try.** Sometimes we trick ourselves into believing our hair is cleaner than it is, spending 15 minutes trying to do something cute, before realising IT'S NOT GONNA WORK and now there's no time. Idiots. Either reset the hair as fast as possible (wet it, mousse it and blow dry some shape into it), add volume powder all over the scalp and pull it up into a messy bun; or comb through a hard, wet-look gel on damp hair then scrape it back, adding big earrings and bright lipstick to distract the masses.

## 3.

**You've washed your hair and need to look groomed but have no time to blow dry.** Great reason to own a product that hastens blow dry time for a smooth result, fast. (I'm fond of Aveda's Smooth Infusion Style Prep Smoother and Kerastase Ciment Thermique.) Apply said product through damp hair before roughly drying hair off. Tie back everything *except* the top layer of hair and fringe. Take a barrel brush and blow dry this top section and fringe/face-framing bits so it's smooth and dry. Shape this smooth top section into an elegant, deep side part and undo your low 'rest of hair' pony, then gather it all together and bun it. Ha! It looks like you blow dried the whole thing! You wizard!

## 5.

**Wear a hat or beanie.** Proceed with caution, though: sombreros are an acquired taste.

# GET SEXY, TEXTURED SECOND-DAY HAIR, INSTANTLY.

So, you've probably seen people like Alexa Chung, Rosie Huntington-Whiteley, the Olsens and pretty much every model in every cool clothing ad campaign ever, and looked at their hair and thought, 'Man, I could really go some nachos right now.' And then, not seconds later, thought, 'How, HOW do they get that gritty, textured, bedhead, matte look? What is the product or the styling step that they know, and I do not? Why is my hair always fluffy or too shiny when sometimes I just want it to be all rock and roll and sexy?'

Here is the answer: Magic dust. Also known as volume, texture or hair powder.

**What it is:** A 'wet' dust. One of the strangest textures I've ever felt. It comes out like powder, but then changes into a kind of...invisible...wet...something. Kind of how I imagine the inside of a frog's house to feel.

**What it does:** Instantly grits up your hair. Gives texture. A dry matte finish. Thickens the hair. Makes it gently piecey, without making it look lank or greasy. Adds volume. Makes clean, slippery hair look second-day. Enthuses people to comment on your hair. Enthuses those same people to be jealous of your hair.

**How you apply it:** Important note: This stuff can only be used on DRY HAIR. Shake a small amount onto your hands if you're a novice. (Stylists will powder it directly onto the scalp. So renegade!) Then rub into the scalp where you want some A) Grit and B) Volume.

**What I do:** On freshly washed, styled hair, that looks… nice… but not sexy and filmclipy, I flip my head over and sprinkle lightly all over the underneath of my hair for a few seconds. I then flip my head up and massage it in. There is INSTANT volume. Amazing. Then, I either sprinkle or rub in from my hands a teeny bit on the top of my scalp/the crown/my fringe area.

YOU MUST GO GENTLY HERE. Like frizz serums, if you put too much in, it's very hard to back up. It becomes concrete-esque. So, just a teeny bit in there, and a bit of a rub and it's done. Another reason to tread lightly is that if you only do a bit, you can add some more tomorrow and keep the style going, whereas if you go too hard, tomorrow it might start shifting out of sexy town, and into lankville. (I also rub some into my mid-lengths to ends for texture. I'm wild like that.)

**Products:** Aveda's Pure Abundance Hair Potion, evo Haze Styling Powder, Schwarzkopf Osis Dust It Mattifying Powder.

If you're serious about sexy second-day hair, you need to get serious about magic dust. Which is a hard sentence to take seriously, but I mean it.

# SLICK AS A RAT WITH A GOLD TOOTH.

You know how in advertisements for ludicrously expensive sunglasses or handbags the model has super mega perfect slick hair, flat on her head and tightly pulled back, and then you try it at home and your hair's all like, 'Oh, *riiiight*, so you spend the last three months trying to rootlift and boost me and glamorously curl me, and now, NOW you thunder in with your fancy paddle brush and want me to lie down flat and flyaway free and smooth as if, as if, I'm some kind of TOY that you can manipulate whenever the mood STRIKES you? Well *SCREW YOU*, sunshine' or something to that effect?

*Well*, I once met a hairstylist who under gunpoint revealed to me how it's done, how the backstage genius hair squad do it, how YOU can do it.

Forget styling it and hairspraying and hairspraying and then hairspraying it some more into place like some form of fool. Cos that's what I was doing and believe me I have *completely* forgotten it.

No, the trick is to **mix styling wax and straightening balm in your hands**, and then comb it through wet hair before styling it into a deep side-parted pony, or centre-part bun.

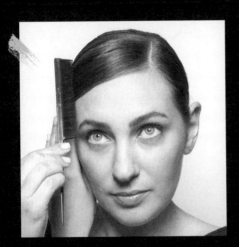

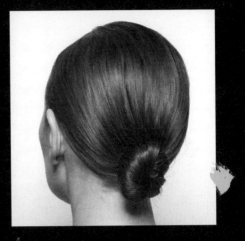

The anonymous hair secret-revealer said hair stylists usually comb it through with a tint brush, as if applying a colour to the hair, but probably we don't own one of those, so we'll just do it with a tailcomb and cheat.

**HERE'S ONE WAY YOU MIGHT LIKE TO SASS YOUR NEW, SLICK HAIR:**

1 Make a perfect part with the skewer end of your tailcomb.

2 Carefully comb the front of your hair so that it's bubble-free and perfect.

3 Tie your hair into a low, slick ponytail, twist into a bun and secure neatly with bobby pins.

4 Smile because you've nailed it.

*Bonus trick!*

*For a slick, chic (but non-greaseball) ponytail, smooth frizzies by gliding a matte hair wax over the top layer of hair before putting it into the elastic.*

# WHEN YOU'RE DOING AN UPDO AT HOME.

**Keep it dirty:** Do not even THINK about THINKING about doing it on clean hair. It must, must be second-day hair. That way you have some grip and texture, instead of stupid, slippery clean hair that won't hold a style and looks nothing like that Kate Bosworth picture you're using as inspiration.

**Mousse control:** Mousse is terrific when you need to Do Something Special with your hair for an event – the trick is to blow dry it through your hair the night before, roughly and half-assedly. Then, the next day, spray through some thermal protectant and style away.

**Spray it:** If you're doing lots of clever bobby pin work, hairspray the pins before you put them in, and gently backcomb the area you're jamming them into too, if possible – keeps them in place.

**Now you do it:** For an elegant, simple and foolproof updo, ensure you have second-day hair, then (1) tong random pieces throughout the hair in every direction and (2) lightly hairspray all over. Next, if possible, dust some hair powder (see page 196) all over the scalp and massage it in for extra grit and texture, then (3) softly scrape it all back into a chignon or a low bun at the base of your neck and (4) pin it loosely, tugging gently at the bun to make it fuller. Pull pieces out around the face or neck if you prefer a softer look (5).

*Remember:*

*If in doubt, spend the time blow drying/styling your hair and wear it out. Updos only look (and feel) right about 50% of the time.*

*Bonus trick!*

*For a fast, polished quiff (delightful with smooth sides and a high pony), use a tailcomb to backcomb sections of the front area (the fringe section), then comb over the big rats' nest you've created gently with the comb and pin into place.*

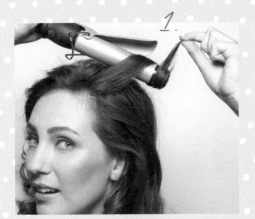

1.

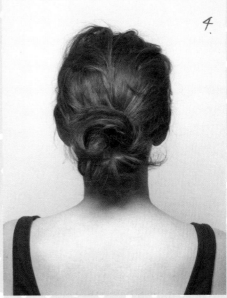

4.

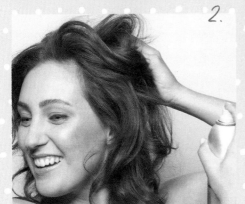

2.

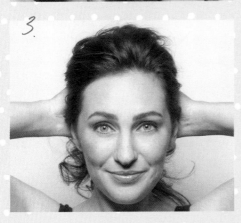

5.

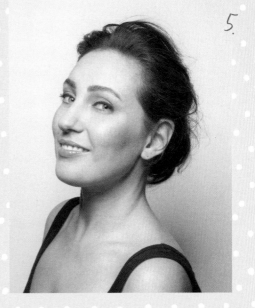

3.

# THE TRICK TO MAKING A PONYTAIL OR TOP KNOT LOOK LIVED-IN AND SEXY: A FUZZY HALO.

I have always struggled with this one, 'this one' being how to make a relatively tight hairstyle look as though I created it yesterday and slept in it, and now I have this adorable little halo of chic fuzz around it that softens the look, and makes it look runway and cool, as opposed to, like, 'I am a ballerina' (who, while extremely talented, tend to wear tight hairstyles that don't flatter 98.6% of the population) or like I stood in front of the mirror and tried to make it look deliberately dishevelled by pulling pieces down around my face, which, as we all know, never works, and looks utterly contrived.

Big difference, isn't there? One is cool and fresh, and one is perfect, tight and 'done'.

So how the heck can a girl get this fuzzy halo? You'll GASP with the simplicity, you really will.

All you need to do is put your hair up as you desire, as tight or as loose as you please, then place the area where your palm and wrist meet on the hair and gently tease it all over the hair. For added sexy dishevely business, tug and pull at the top knot or bun or pony to make it look a bit scruffier too.

**HERE'S A VISUAL STEP-BY-STEP SO YOU GET THE IDEA:**

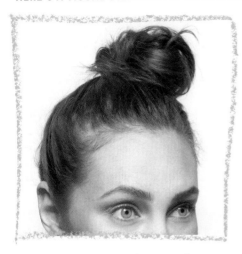

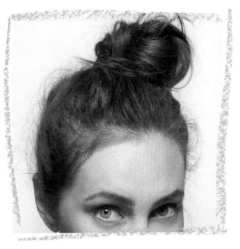

**1** The high messy bun is created in around two seconds.

See?! Much better. Makes what can appear too 'done' instantly more modern and fresher.

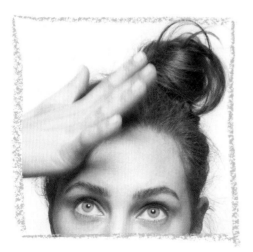

*Pay heed or stuff it up, dumdum!*

- *Hair must be perfectly dry for this to work. Preferably a bit dirty too.*

- *Leave it fluffy at the end of your palm teasing. Do NOT spray hairspray, or shine mist, or Mortein or anything on the hair once you're done. Leave it well alone.*

- *The fuzzy halo is the perfect way to un-perfect a really pretty or feminine dress or outfit. Too-neat hair with super-pretty clothes is too thematic.*

**2** The palm/wrist area is used to gently rub and tease the hair all over the head.

**3** The bun is tugged at gently to match the fuzzy halo on the rest of the head.

# CHANGING THE PART IN YOUR HAIR CAN MAKE YOU 453 TIMES SEXIER.

If you know which side of your face is 'most attractive' (stronger, more photogenic), you can figure out where it is best to part your hair, which serves to amplify that attractiveness. Donald Trump has been using this to great effect for decades.

**To find out which is your stronger side:** Pull all your hair back and up and look for one side of your face to be more square in the jaw line area (stronger) and the other to be more curved (softer).

In my case, the strong side was SO STINKIN' OBVIOUS. When I parted my hair so that the fringe and front layers obscured the left side of my face, my cheekbones looked way more angular than they actually are, my eyes were more prominent (all of the 'angles' appear to push your eyes forward) and my jaw line more pronounced.

When I flipped my fringe over to the other, 'soft' side, my face didn't look so angular and, well, nice. Was puffy in contrast.

Try it yourself, you'll see. (You might already intrinsically know which is your strong side, because it will often be the side you tilt your face for photos/selfies.)

**Fun fact that is a bit politically incorrect!**
A side-part (on the strong side) is apparently the
hairstyle men find the most attractive because by having
one eye partially covered, you draw all the attention to
your lovely angular cheekbone and your jaw line and
your lips.

This makes sense when you consider that body
language-wise, one of the most common and
subconscious things women do to look more attractive
to the opposite sex is to pull back the hair from one side
of our neck and tuck it behind our ear, so that we A)
expose all that lovely neck skin, B) show off our lovely
jawline, and C) open up that whole area, which makes
it – and us – look inviting.

So, as Shakespeare once famously said: 'Flip your
part and suddenly be all alluring and cheekbony and
photogenic and feminine and shit!'

# A SEXY FACE-COVERING CENTRE PART IS ALWAYS IN FASHION.

You know the one. It's like you're peeking through little hair curtains, because the fringe/front layers of your hair are falling down lazily over your eyes. It's very sexy, wouldn't you agree? Very French and mysterious and alluring, like you're playing some kind of sexy hide and seek, without actually having to squeeze into a dark wardrobe.

When it comes to creating this look, it's all about the front section. And the fact that the hair has been styled *forward*, not *back*.

YOU NEED:

• Clean, wet hair

• Mousse

• Thermal protectant spray

• A mid-sized barrel brush

• A comb

• Blow-dryer with nozzle attachment on

• Sectioning clips/butterfly clips

• Some 'magic dust' (see page 196)

• Some biscuits in case you get hungry

**YOU DO THIS:**

**1** Run a golf-ball size amount of mousse through your hair; tips, midlengths, roots: all of it. Spray lightly all over with a thermal protectant spray.

**2** Comb through.

**3** Section all hair up and away from the crown/fringe/hairline, leaving a good two inches out all around the face. Obviously this style works better if you have long front layers, or no front layers and all-one-length hair. Shorter fringes will ruin the line of the hair. Incredibly inconsiderate.

**4** Begin blow drying the front section STRAIGHT DOWN over the face on high heat, going over each section again and again, just like in the salon. You will look like Cousin It for this part. It will be highly comical. Take tiny sections so you're thorough. This is especially important if you have cowlicks or curls.

**5** Also blow dry both sides of the front in the opposite direction to how it normally sits; this will iron out kinks. Make sure you do it for the hair on the sides as well as on top. When it's dry, gently move it into a centre-part, and on a lower power, blow dry it into this part. Doesn't need to be perfect, you'll go over it again at the end. It's just crucial to style this part when the hair is wet, is all.

**6** Blow dry the rest of the hair, actively blow drying it all forward towards the face.

**7** Once all hair is done, go over the front section again, styling it into an almost vertical centre-part, bringing in the weight from the rest of your hair to further bring it forward, and pointing the nozzle of the hair dryer down the hair so it's smooth. Set with a blast of cold air for 60 seconds. *Important*.

**8** Use a small amount of polishing serum, hairspray or magic dust (see page 196) through the mid-lengths to ends for a bit of movement and piecey-ness.

**9** Peer sexily through your fancy hair curtains and wink at a stranger or two.

# FIVE
## ways to make your hair look longer.

I recently had a haircut where I walked away with longer (looking) hair. There were no extensions or wizards involved, just a clever peanut who knew I was trying to grow my hair, and understood my one-length blunt bob would need to quietly leave. Here's the trickery I utilise when I am in the frustrating grow-y-out phase:

## 2.

**The styling.** If you've ever had your hair loosely curled in-salon and wondered why it looks longer than when *you* do it, I'll reveal the mystery: black magic. Just kidding: it's about the ends. Pros often leave a few centimetres straight at the end of their waves, which creates an optical illusion of the hair being longer. To DIY, just leave a few cm out of your styler/tongs when you style it.

## 1.

**The haircut.** When you sit down, ask your cutter for a cut/trim that will make your hair look longer. They will laugh. Ignore them. Usually this entails blended layers that will make your hair look *flowier*, as opposed to a blunt style. Definitely use hair masks and treatments, and, despite it feeling counterintuitive, have trims every six weeks – split ends won't add to lengthy lusciousness, they will stagnate your style, and look lank and brittle.

**4.**

**The texture.** Straight hair looks longer than curly hair, but I tend to think the wave with the straight ends as detailed in #2 makes hair look *even longer*. Add some beach spray to the mid-lengths, and hair powder at the roots for a bit of volume and movement.

**3.**

**The part.** For reasons unknown to everyone, a middle part will make your hair look longer. Which is a shame if your hair is teaming with cowlicks, or is cut to a side part. But it's worth investigating, so do the trick on page 195, before butterfly-clipping (bobby pins leave dents) each side down near your ears so the hair sets/cools into the centre part. Apply your makeup/shine your shoes/ feed your goats, then release the clips and enjoy!

**5.**

**Wear a wig.** A long one, you doofus!

# FAKE CASUAL HAIR EVEN IF IT'S UPTIGHT AND REALLY CLEAN.

You don't win friends with superclean, fluffy hair, and that's a fact. No, you win them by having a swimming pool.

Or hair that tells the world you're too cool to care and you may not ever wash it or style it, because it is inherently great. This is anti-hairdressing hair. Dirty looking, matte, dishevelled, bedhead hair. It's not clean, or polished or neat. But it IS sexy and messy.

1 Don't use conditioner. If your hair can take it, leaving it a bit rougher and without the heavy coat of conditioner will grant you instant cool girl texture.

2 Seasalt spray. Spray it all through damp (or even dry!) hair, then blast your hair dryer on high heat all over for 30 seconds. Instant texture and grip and grit, whether you leave it out or do a messy pony/bun.

3 Spray any kind of texture/beach spray onto damp hair, twist it up into a high bun and secure. Blow dry the bun for a few minutes, then release and finger comb. Use volume powder/hair dust all over to finish.

# RICH WOMAN IN WINTER HAIR.

Picture a woman in a camel-coloured skivvy, sitting by a fire, sipping a blood-coloured merlot and talking about the origins of Greek Philosophy or handbags, I can never remember which. She's wearing soft brown shadow and a taupe lipstick, but the HAIR, dear GOD her HAIR! It is stupendous! So long, so shiny, so healthy, so smooth! It's as though she's never been outside or seen a blow-dryer in her life.

I call this Rich Woman in Winter hair. It's luxuriously soft, rich-looking hair, side-parted and posh, beautifully bouncy and shiny and falling languorously. It is extremely polished. Chic. *Expensive*.

And, provided you have hair that is longer than your chin, getting this look is achievable!

- As you know by now, first run mousse through hair and mist some thermal protectant through.

- Blow dry it smooth with a large vented barrel brush to straighten it out but give body, and then go over the hair with a paddle brush misted with hairspray for a super-smooth finish. Finish with a blast of cold air to set. No stylers or irons, please.

- A slight kick at the ends is perfectly acceptable because we quite like the bounce, thank you.

- Add a Rolls-Royce and a ridiculous purebred dog that is incredibly unattractive despite costing a shittonne of money, and you're done.

# HOW TO STYLE A SHORT FRINGE.

1 Apply a whisper of product to tame frizz, assist with shaping and hold, and protect against heat styling.

2 Blow dry hair using a small barrel brush firmly across both sides of the forehead so that all cowlicks are tamed and fringe is full and well-behaved.

3 Gently style/flat-iron the fringe down (on low heat, if, say, you own a styler with that option), shaping it so it sits naturally against the shape of the head. (Use the trick on page 185.)

4 Slick back and hairspray into place the little fuzzy wings either side of the fringe. (A toothbrush is excellent for this.)

5 Lightly mist with a setting hairspray to make it behave for many hours.

6 Ponder whether you might grow it out eventually.

7 Naaaahh.

**Short fringes look great on:** long or heart-shaped faces, while wispy eye-skimmers better suit rounder face shapes. If you have an oval face, you can have whatever the heck fringe you want. (And if you have cowlicks, curls or the unsightly 'middle-part', blow dry your fringe as normal, then point the nozzle of your hair dryer down the fringe and set it to cold. This will set it, and make it all shiny and impressive. Alternatively, consider having the fringe section keratin-smoothed.)

# SHOW YOUR COWLICKS WHO IS BOSS. (HINT: YOU.)

*Bonus trick!*
*Spray hairspray onto a toothbrush and use on baby hairs or those annoying frizzy bits around the face to smooth them down real flat and real good.*

As my hair is the CEO of the Independent United Cowlick's Front, it refuses to entertain a fringe, or to do a convincing centre-part. In fact, it barely offers a semi-centre-part that will give me a headache when my hair is permitted to return to its natural, bovine-saliva-drenched state.

And that's when it's *styled!* When there are tools and power points available! But so often there are not. And the humidity is stronger than a jug of Absinthe. And I'm mid-way through the day and it's drizzling, and need help to control my fringe from curling up or sitting flat and stupid.

**SO HERE'S WHAT I DO.**

• When I'm sitting at my desk or getting ready to go out *or even in the taxi,* I flip my part over to the irregular side of my forehead, that is, the side I never, ever part it, because it looks wrong and is going against 456 cowlicks and potentially some very aggressive curls, and I hold it there for as long as possible. Bobby pin it if I can. Hairspray it too, if I can.

• Then, when it's time to roll, I shake out my hair, part it in the middle and, hovering hairpins, it *behaves!* And it always does, when I do this. *You gotta try it out and see!* Just try it and see.

# REGARDING YOUR LOVE AFFAIR WITH DRY SHAMPOO...

Because we all have one by now, obviously, since dry shampoo (actually a finely textured powder in an aerosol can and not really a shampoo at all) is one of the greatest hair products since Celia Von Barrelsworth invented hair itself in 1907.

**HERE'S A QUICK GUIDE TO DRY SHAMPOO THAT IS ACTUALLY PRETTY SLOW:**

**Dry shampoo saves your ass when your hair is filthy or you are running late or you wish to extend your blow dry** for another day because it instantly soaks up all the grease and oil on your scalp, giving you nice, clean-looking hair again.

**Dry shampoo is also a terrific styling product**. Spray it into freshly washed hair, in stripes going along the scalp, lifting up sections of hair as you go, for a lovely matte texture. Also gives volume.

Dry shampoos that are actually more like coloured, wet paint (I'm talking to you, Bumble & bumble) **are wonderful for covering up roots** that need doing. Be sparing with these ones, though, as you really only get one day of application out of them. So, uh, wait till your hair is truly filthy, is the message.

Dry shampoo in a travel size (Batiste does one) is pretty much **the most important thing you can put into your gym bag**. Spray all over and rub in with your fingers to soak up any sweat and oil that accumulated as you spun on a stationary bike like a crazed demon on 12 Red Bulls.

**The less you can spray on the actual top of your scalp, where it's visible, the better**. (Go under that layer instead; flip the head upside down too if you want all-over freshness.) After one application you get a lovely, dry, soaked-up-grease finish. After two or three days (very common for me) it starts to build up and look a little bit like dandruff. Sexy.

**Dry shampoo, like any hair product, builds up over time**. And if you're only shampooing your hair once each wash (we talked about this on page 175), there's very little chance you're actually removing all of that powder you keep spraying in. So, consider switching to a detox or clarifying shampoo. (Especially if you also love the hair dust/powder and texturising creams like I do.) GO EASY with these clarifying shampoos if you have coloured hair, though, because these products sometimes fade that lovely colour.

If you're in a real pickle (as opposed to a pretend one, made of plastic or something) **you can use a bit of baby powder instead**. A lot of session stylists (people who style hair for magazine fashion spreads or advertising campaigns) still do, and may never switch to the stuff in a can because they are purists and the talc works better and so on and so forth. Whatever lifts your luggage, I say.

# HOW TO HAVE GOOD HAIR AFTER SMASHING THE TREADMILL.

1 Pack dry shampoo, elastics, bobby pins, shower cap (and a small barrel brush if you have fierce cowlicks) in your gym bag.

2 Before you start honing your guns, pull your hair up loosely, so as not to ruin the 'style' you've got going. This is especially crucial for curly hair, or nicely blow-dried hair. Too tight will wreck things. Sort out loose annoying or fringey bits with bobby pins, and always, always have surplus amounts of both elastics and these wily little devils in your gym bag.

3 Wear a shower cap in the shower. Once out, crack out the dry shampoo. See how the other girls in the change room envy you with your shiny can of magic. *Clever you.*

4 Flip your head upside down and spray dry shampoo quickly all over, then flip back up and spray around your hairline and quickly along the scalp. Massage it in so it soaks up the dampness.

5 If possible, now blast your hair with a blow-dryer on high heat (or use the hand-dryer). If you have cowlicks or your hair has gone wrongly, use a smallish barrel brush to style it.

6 *Well.* This is nice. You deserve to look pretty for doing something so sweaty, dull and time-consumey, and now you do.

# WHICH HAIRSTYLE FOR WHICH OCCASION?

Terrific question.

**If you're on a first date** – wear your hair out. It's annoying and sexist (and, some say, a case of biological predisposition towards women who look young and in good health, of which healthy, shiny hair supposedly symbolises) but it's often how we feel our most attractive/confident.

**If you're wearing a very elaborate dress with lots going on, a high collar, or striking neck jewellery** – wear your hair up or back. Keep the focus on the dress, necklace or face.

**If you're wearing a very simple black dress** – do something exciting with your hair, whether that is textured, sexy waves with a centre-part, or Veronica Lake style vintage waves that are perfectly tonged, brushed out and sprayed into place, or a sexy, scruffy ponytail. In a nutshell – your dress is simple, try not to let your hair (or makeup) be.

**If you're going to a ball and have zero time** – wet your hair under the shower, but don't wash it. Now comb through either straightening balm, gel or even hairspray with a fine-tooth comb. Create a deep side-part, and comb it all down and back into a low, tight bun. Don't spray again as it will look too helmet – it should look wet and slick, not hard and crunchy. (See page 198 for the full how-to.)

**If you're at the beach and are off to lunch or drinks** – embrace the texture and muss it up even more, or if you have long hair, do a deep side part and pull the length around over one shoulder and plait it, or pull it up high into a messy top knot and pop in some big, rowdy earrings.

**If you're wanting to be taken 'seriously'** – wear your hair either polished and blow-dried, or back in a very neat fashion. Nothing edgy, wild, scruffy or top-knotty, probably.

**If you're wanting to be taken 'not seriously'** – wear a hat in the shape of an ice-cream cone, and a thick handlebar moustache.

# LEAVE A FACIAL WITHOUT THE WORST HAIR IN THE UNIVERSE.

When one has a facial, one is very, very likely to come out of said facial with oily roots, lankness and a greasiness that WILL NOT GO AWAY, no matter how much styling you attempt.

But there's a way around it. Just follow the rules of Post-Facial Rubbish Hair Avoidance, you turkey!

### THE RULES OF POST-FACIAL RUBBISH HAIR AVOIDANCE.

**Do this:** Take a bobby pin and a hair band, and get that hair into a very high pony or loose bun, and get that fringe well, well away.

**Say this:** 'Um ... I've actually got to go to lunch/dinner/a date/a job interview/ my wedding after this, and so I was hoping to keep my hair fresh? Is it possible for you to not massage my scalp and pop a headband on to keep the products away from my hair? Thanks sooo much. I really appreciate it. So sorry to be a pain in the arse.'

**Why you need to say that, and in that way:** Most therapists are very good at what they do. They are highly trained, and they don't like to be told how to do their thing (and lots of facials involve the kind of massage that results in oily hair). Which is fair – do they come in and tell you how to wash your donkeys? (Look, I know you're a donkey washer. Don't be ashamed. It's okay. Your mum told me.) So by asking her to avoid your hairline and scalp in a sweet, non passive-aggressive manner, she will take extra care to avoid ruining your mop, while still endeavouring to give you the best dingin' facial you've ever known.

And that's nice, I think.

Of course, the Very Smart thing to do is book your facial at the end of the day when you can just roll home and not even think about makeup or having to have pretty hair. Just like that old Beethoven song: 'I gots the greasiest of hair, and I jus' don' care.' (At the very least wear a hat to your appointment so you can continue your day without showing off your greasy hair and red face.)

*Bonus trick!*

*Need great skin for an event? Omnilux and oxygen-infusions aside, always get a facial (at least) the day/night before, not the day of.*

*Bonus trick!*

*Your best reactive chance against catastrophic post-facial hair is to either use some dry shampoo/talc and change your part (freshens the hair immediately) or create a very slick and wet-looking low bun or pony.*

# HOW TO ELEGANTLY TELL YOUR HAIRDRESSER YOU REALLY DISLIKE YOUR HAIR COLOUR.

You've just spent two hours having a colour done but at the end of the dry and style, you realise you'd rather eat toenail clippings than be stuck with it for five minutes, let alone five months. It's GROSS.

Unbelievably, you're probably going to pay and leave without saying a word about your misery. I know many, manymanymany women who are Total Grown Ups and very powerful and assertive day to day, but who turn into lambs in the hair chair.

But *you must say something*. You must!

The salon and colourist **do not benefit** from you hating your colour and potentially spreading the word of how unhappy you were with their service. They would much prefer you to leave happy. Or at least with an appointment to remedy the situation.

**It's your hair**. You wear it every day. It's your best accessory and mood-maker. *You need to love it.*

**HERE'S HOW TO PLAY IT:**

**1** Most of the drama can be avoided before the dye is applied by **having a FULL consultation with your colourist before she or he begins**. Take photos of the colour you want. Ask to see the swatches from the colour they'll mix up. Say things like, 'So, it will be how much darker/lighter than my current colour?' and 'Is there any chance the dye will come out lighter or darker than we think?' and 'I'm terrified of it coming out too dark/making my skin tone look washed out/the highlights looking really obvious. That won't happen, will it?' so that you have a full understanding of the risks, and she/he knows what you're scared of, and will avoid it.

**2** **Should you be unhappy at the end refer to this consultation**, as it gives you a simple, non-emotional reference point. You might say, 'Oooh, I thought we said it wouldn't be more than a shade or two darker than my previous colour . . . but I think that's definitely too dark. Is there any way we can remedy this easily?' Which keeps things nice, and helps sort out what the issue is, and who was at fault.

**3** Be honest and human and take some responsibility (even if deep down you don't think you're at fault) rather than being scary and aggressive and bitchy. **Everyone makes mistakes and hair dye reacts differently on everyone's hair depending on the condition of it and the base colour** etc. Chances are your colourist knows it doesn't look that great too and, if you are kind, will be more than accommodating in fixing it. Say things like, 'I am really, really sorry, but I just didn't expect it to look like this . . . I probably explained myself badly. Is there any way at all we can fix this?'

**4** If your consultation was thorough and you have images that were the reference and your hair looks completely different, you have a good case for getting the fix for free. But if your colourist didn't have a clear idea of what you wanted, and did what they thought you wanted and you hate it, you may have to pay. Ask if there's any chance for a discount at the least. **And BE NICE**. Much more likely to get a favourable outcome if you remain friendly. That goes for everything in life, actually.

**5** In the WCS, if your colourist or the salon is being unhelpful, and you have been lovely but feel you were definitely in the right, and they refuse to fix it unless you pay full price, **consider a salon switch**. It's an area that is rife with error and miscalculations and subjectivity and if you and your colourist or salon can't come to some kind of meet-halfway agreement, you might be happier at another salon.

**6** Try not to roast them on social media, even though it's tempting. Instead, send in your bikie boyfriend, Booger, and get *him* to sort things out for you.

# HANDS
# +
# NAILS

When my nails are chipped or too
long, I feel grubby and unprepared.
But when they're nicely manicured,
I feel glamorous and polished, like
I can take on the world, one daintily
held glass of Fanta at a time.

So come on!
Let's pull our fingers out!
Get a hand on the situation!
Really nail it!
Etc.

# THE INTERNATIONAL ASSOCIATION FOR REAL NICE LOOKING NAILS PRESENTS, NAIL RULES, THE UPDATED VERSION.

1 Long nails are rarely considered to be very attractive or elegant, despite what Rihanna would have you believe. The most alluring length is a few millimetres above the tip of the finger.

2 If you are wearing a very dark polish, keep your nails short, neat and square with slightly rounded edges.

3 If you are wearing a jovial pink, orange, jade, blue or coral, you can afford to have your nails a touch longer than when wearing dark shades.

4 If you are having a French manicure or pedicure, insist that the white line across the top is *very thin*. It's meant to mimic the natural overspill of your nail on top of your skin, and because we know that overspill is quite diminutive, so too should that white strip be.

5 If you insist on having acrylic nails, this does not give you licence to have Very Long Nails. In fact, the only way to remain looking chic with acrylic nails is to keep them an elegant, shortish length.

6 For a timeless ladylike look, have your nails shaped into ovals, and then paint them crimson or fire engine red, or even plum.

7 For a swell look guaranteed to make people dizzy with envy (or just dizzy), substitute liquid paper for polish. (This is a joke. Obviously.)

# TWO THIN,

# NOT ONE THICK.

*Bonus trick!*
*If you don't have a nail file but DO have an annoying nail jag – use the side of a box of matches.*

You may have read somewhere once (*definitely not in this book*) that if you must get out the door but NEED to have pretty nails, one thick coat of polish slapped onto your talons will do the trick. I am here to say that this is an utter falsity, because how can putting a **thick** glob of something that already takes time to dry, even when spread **thin**, be a clever idea?

It can't be.

It's silly and we must all do our best to stop these dreadful lies once and for all.

What *must* be done are *two very speedy thin layers.*

Give each layer 60 seconds to dry and you'll be a lot happier when just 15 minutes later you need to dig into your handbag for your keys, trust me.

Of course, there is a whole market of quick-dry polishes that dry in 1.4 seconds and require one speedy coat of polish and they are perfect for these situations. However. While this breed of polish is ideal for holy-shit-I-need-to-have-nice-nails-to-meet-his-mother-because-she-is-always-immaculately-groomed-to-the-point-where-I-feel-inadequate-but-that-is-PROBABLY-THE-POINT, it is most definitely *unideal* for long-term gratification because they'll chip in a day or two.

But use them as intended – as a stopgap polish application – and you'll be happy. Most are even so kind as to have a brush that is particularly easy to use, which ensures that even someone who has just drunk three double espressos can achieve a slick mani in minutes.

# CHOOSE A DELIGHTFULLY FLATTERING POLISH FOR YOUR SKIN TONE.

**IF YOU CAN'T BE BOTHERED READING THIS PAGE, STICK TO THIS RULE:**

Choose nail polish colours in the same shades as lipsticks that flatter your lips.

**IF YOU CAN BE BOTHERED READING THIS PAGE:**

**Fair Skin:**
**Yes!** Soft pink as well as blue-based lacquers in berry colours like strawberry, cranberry or raspberry. (Try OPI That's Berry Daring.)

**Not so much...** Flesh and light candy-colour tones will drain the life out of your hands.

**Medium skin:**
**Yes!** Burgundies, plums and wine tones: win. Bright shades like orange and fuchsia will make skin appear more tanned; pastels and sorbet tones paler. (Try Essie Bahama Mama.)

**Not so much...** Dark navy and black.

**Olive skin:**
**Yes!** Bright and tropical shades like orange, tangerine, coral and melon and hot pink look TERRIFIC, so too browns, taupe and brick-reds. (Try Orly Truly Tangerine.)

**Not so much...**
Golds.

**Dark skin:**
**Yes!** Go dark and strong, you vampy varnish vixen. Powerful reds, deep purples, blacks, bronze, greens – the world is your nail salon. Almond and caramel-based nudes also look frightfully good. (Try OPI Going My Way or Norway.)

**Not so much...** Whites, pearlescent pastels and silvers.

*Bonus tip!*
*If your dress and hair and makeup and shoes and bag are as sweet as a sugar sachet covered in honey, go for black, dark violet or blood red nails.. So surprising! So jarring! So confusing! So avant garde! So talking-pointy!*

# A LIST OF CLEVER THINGS YOU CAN DO TO MAKE NAIL POLISH APPLICATION LOOK GOOD AND DRY FAST:

• If you've been exfoliating or pushing down or clipping your cuticles, take a cotton pad and apply polish remover to your nails again before polishing. Oils or moisturisers on the nails will make varnish behave in an extremely disobedient fashion.

• Always use a base coat, even if your manicurist says you don't need one because it's a light shade. She should know better.

• If you have an uneven nail surface, apply a ridge-filler and base coat in one so you have a smooth canvas.

• To make varnish last, run the polish brush *horizontally along the actual tip of each nail* as well as the nail bed, so that you're basically painting the underside. This 'locks in' the polish.

• If you don't have top coat, drip cuticle oil over the nails to speed up drying time.

• Use a quick-dry drip over the top, ensuring you leave 60 seconds between top coat and doing this. But only if you really need your nails to dry fast – quick-dry products can disrupt the polish/top coat.

• To clean up your errors (applying after whisky again, were we?), wait till the polish is *thoroughly dry*, then dip an eye-shadow applicator in polish remover to clean up the skin around the nail.

• A thick, high-shine top coat will hide errors and smudges. Try: Sally Hansen MegaShine.

• Don't jam your hands in front of a fan to dry them, it just causes air bubbles.

• Do your nails at your desk and let them dry as you faff about on Facebook and pretend to work.

*Bonus trick!*
*Make your nail polish last twice as long by doing proper prep before painting (totally clean, polish- and moisturiser-free nails and a layer of base coat) and applying a top coat every second day.*

# YOUR HANDS WILL MAKE YOU APPEAR OLDER THAN YOU ARE.

All that money you're spending on your skin care to look 25 **doesn't matter** when your hands make you look 45.

Hands are extremely susceptible to ageing and, in a real blow to hand lovers, usually age faster than any other area on your body.

**Why:** The skin is so thin! There's hardly any flesh or fat on the back of your hand, so when the collagen or elastin fibres break down due to ageing, you get wrinkly, crepe-like skin and your veins peek through.

Your hands do a lot of things. We wash up with them which zaps moisture; we type and text for hours with them which means sore muscles; and we perform spirit fingers when we're drunk which is embarrassing for them.

We neglect to protect them from the sun – especially when driving, leaving them wide open to UV damage, which brings on sun spots, pigmentation and wrinkles.

**So, LOVE THEM, man!**

- Wear gloves when doing hand washing, washing up, car washing, dog washing, yacht washing...

- Keep hand cream by every sink and moisturise every time you wash your hands. Every time!

- Buy handcream with SPF 30 and keep it in your handbag so that you're protected when outdoors/driving/everyday/always.

- Use leftover face cream on the backs of your hands.

# ACTION REQUIRED: ANTI-AGEING FOR YOUR HANDS.

If you *really* want to fool the public into thinking you're as young as a springtime foal, do what you do to your face to your neck, chest and hands as well – and that means prevention, protection and rejuvenation.

**Easy option that costs very little:** Buy a tube of hand cream with UVA/UVB sunscreen and anti-ageing ingredients like vitamin E and carry it in your handbag... Why do you think it's called a HANDbag! Ha ha ha! Great work, Fosters!

**A little more effort, a better pay-off:** Exfoliate your hands once a week, using a grainy exfoliant to get rid of dead skin cells. Follow with a facemask for 10 minutes.

**Hardest and most expensive with the best pay-off:** Get some photo-rejuvenation, either with IPL (Intense Pulse Light) or a skin retexturising laser like Fraxel.

**Say NO to UV gel polish dryers:** They're like teeny little tanning beds, you dingus! Studies are now linking UV nail-dryers to a rise in the number of cases of skin cancer on the fingers. (All that driving without sunscreen doesn't help, either.) Salons should be using LED lamps to set gel polish now anyway.

# NO, I DON'T SMOKE. WHY DO YOU ASK?

If you're anything like me, you find yourself sporting **yellowed nails and cuticles** far too often.

This is not because you are cool and tough and smoke heaps of ciggies behind the dunnies after school, but because you apply fake tan and don't scrub your hands well enough afterwards. And so you are punished.

**Here is how to remove the evidence:**

1 Wear a tanning mit and don't stain your hands or nails in the first place. (I swear by my Vita Liberata one.)

2 Get an old toothbrush and slather it with whitening toothpaste, and then scrub your fingers and nails with it.

# MAKE AN EFFORT IN YOUR HOLIDAY PHOTOS.

I strenuously salute and encourage a casual attitude to makeup and hair while on a summer holiday.

*However.*

I don't think you should flick off your grooming switch entirely...Rather, I enthuse a brand of glamour that's easy, but gives some real KICK KICK BANG BANG.

**Here's why:**

- It's fun and simple and requires very little work and cost, so pipe down.

- Being on vacation doesn't give you a free pass to walk around looking like you don't give a toot. You're on holidays, darling heart, not invisible!

- Holidays are when we have the most photos taken of us, when we furiously collect memories. When else will you swim off rocks in Croatia? Or drink Campari in Sicily at sunset?

Perhaps never. And yet, so often when we have holiday snaps taken, we're wearing Daggy Holiday Clothes (old sundresses, unflattering shorts, dull tees) that don't do the trip/your happiness/the location justice.

To me it seems unfair that we look great each day for *work*, but when we're in pretty places with people we love and everything is a photo opp, we're wearing a singlet with an olive-oil stain on it, Converse and a cap.

Now, I don't want to come off as a vanity warden who bullies you into thinking you need full makeup and perfect hair when you're schlepping through the streets of Phuket. That is so far from my point it doesn't even *recognise* the point cos it's from another solar system where points don't exist. What I'm saying is that even if all you'll be doing is beach-eat-nap, you can still look lovely.

This was confirmed for me after holidaying with a friend. She packed a straw hat, big black Famous Person sunglasses to conceal hangovers, a few summer scarves, huge decorative earrings and necklaces, some classic and colourful dresses, and a few pairs of sandals. She wore BB cream and lipstick/gloss through the day, and at night slicked her hair back and added some liner and shadow. It took her no time, and she always looked turbo chic, which is about five times more chic than standard chic.

So, I started to, um, copy her.

Consequently our photos from this trip – and we got plenty – are some of my favourite holiday snaps. THEY will be the ones I will show my kids to prove I was a cool travelling babe before I became the tracksuited disciplinarian they know and love.

So! Next time you're off to Bali/Byron/ Barbados, why not wear red lipstick with a wide-brimmed hat and a white shirtdress? Why not add some fun earrings or a necklace from Topshop to a slicked back ponytail? Why not pull your hair into a low braid and snake it down one shoulder, instead of jamming it back? Bold accessories can make any boring black dress exciting, and some simple hair, bronzer and a few coloured lip products should be your holiday BFFs . . . *not* Gary and Shelley from Arizona, despite their best efforts.

Adopting a glamorous holiday persona (I call mine Blanchie) (really!) is fun and easy. You get to sashay through your holiday feeling like a movie star, and then look at your photos knowing you looked pretty great, actually. Because you did! You really did. I saw you. You did.

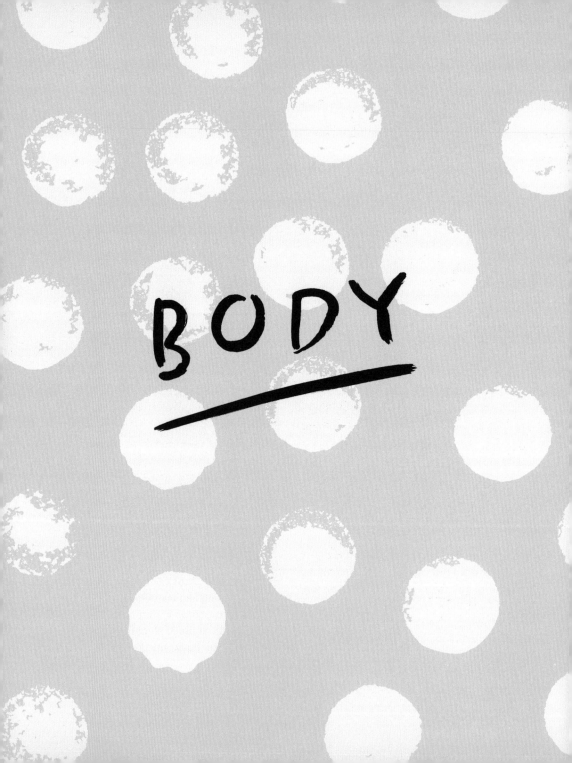

BODY

Despite allowing us to do all kinds of marvellous things, like rollerblade and climb trees in search of sloths, the body is terribly neglected, compared to that fancy pampered guy sitting on top of the neck.

This ends here. TODAY.

The body is covered in skin too, you know! And it's highly visible for many months of the year and it deserves to be cared for and loved and nourished too.

*Written and spoken by the Minister for the Party of Fair Treatment of Bodies.*

# BEAT IT, LITTLE PIMPLE-LIKE BUMPS.

**Little pimple-like bumps:** Usually but not always keratosis pilaris (KP), these little bastards are generally genetic, are caused by blocked or clogged hair follicles, and look like a rash of small red bumps and usually show up on the backs of arms, legs, thighs and the *bum*. The bum!

**Treatment:** It's a REAL good idea to seek professional advice for KP before starting any routine. However, I have been advised by proper doctory people that this is generally what would be prescribed as treatment: a mild exfoliating product, then a gentle body wash for sensitive skin, followed with a body lotion containing AHAs, which will gently exfoliate the skin and encourage new, clear skin cells to come through.

**HERE ARE SOME SUGGESTIONS:**

**First gently exfoliate the area (no harsh scrubs or rough loofahs, you sweet dunce!)** with a cotton face cloth or a gentle sugar oil–based scrub, or by using a dry body brush before your shower.

**Then wash your skin with something nourishing and sensitive** like MooGoo Milk Soap or Cetaphil Gentle Skin Cleanser.

**Then apply a moisturising cream with AHAs** and slather it all over. You could try MD Formulations Hand & Body Creme, NeoStrata Ultra Smoothing Lotion 10% AHA, or Palmers Anti-Aging Smoothing Lotion.

**Additional trick for no extra cost:** Use pawpaw ointment on *very* unhappy red/bumpy areas before showering to prevent the area getting irritated and dried out. Also, take vitamin E. It helps. If you are getting no relief, if might be worth investigating microdermabrasion.

# SAY YOU HAVE SOME PIMPLES ON YOUR CHEST...

And it's too late to change your outfit, or you just don't want to change your outfit because it's positively scorchy, so you do what any woman would do, and crack out your concealer and try to cover them up, just as you would a spot on your face.

*Wrong*. These are not spots on your face. And they are not your under-eye area. These are spots on your chest. And they require their own special treatment.

1 Buy a concealer palette – you get a variety of concealer shades which you can blend for different areas of the face and body or skin tone, according to your tan/the season. Napoleon Perdis does one, and I sincerely wish more brands would, for they are terrific.

2 Mix a little bit of foundation with some creamy concealer a shade darker than your face. (Or lighter, depending on the colour of your chest.)

3 Using a very pointed, thin brush, apply the tiniest bit of your potion onto the spot. And keep it very, very targeted on the spot. Do not blend it out a few centimetres each way because A) that is a moronic idea and B) it makes it very obvious you are trying to conceal something.

4 Set it with a dot of powder and get on with your night already, you sizzling little sausage.

# HEY I KNOW YOU'RE COLD, BUT THAT'S NO EXCUSE TO BE SCALY TOO.

*Bonus trick!*
*If your body butter is too thick, but you need and want the extra moisture for your skin, scoop out a bit of the body butter and pour some or jojoba or coconut oil into the container to give it more spread.*

I also know that standing on cold tiles on a morning that's as cold as balls after your shower and putting on body lotion is about as enticing as a warm mussel milkshake. *But*. There *are* ways to not freeze your kicker off and remain scale-free.

1 Don't even think about using body lotion that isn't in a pump or spray form. They make everything so much easier.

   **Such as:** Dove Summer Glow (for those addicted to their tan), Dermalogica Body Hydrating Cream, Vaseline Intensive Care Spray and Go.

2 Kick the lotion habit altogether and use an in-shower oil. Body cleansing oils clean the skin without stripping it of much-needed oils and often negate the need for a body moisturiser afterwards.

   **Products:** Nutrimetics Nutri-Rich Shower Oil, Kiehl's Superbly Restorative Argan Body Cleansing Oil, Palmer's Skin Therapy Oil.

3 Actually, there is no three. Well I'm sorry! GOD, you're so *demanding* these days! It never used to be like this. You've changed.

   *sobs*

   *remembers hates these asterisk aside things*

   *wonders what else can use to express emotions or actions*

   +these are no good+

   <or these>

   %these are terrible%

   *guess it's back to these*

# SCRUB OUT OF THE TUB.

Ever glance down at your legs and think, gosh, I should really use a body scrub cos my skin feels a bit rough and some exfoliation would be a splendid thing to do to get me soft and lovely again and ohgoodLORD *look at those fake tan streaks on my ankles!* How was I walking around like that and NOBODY TOLD ME? I feel like a stripy little *fool!* Like an orange-ankled little *twit!*… and so on and so forth and that kind of caper.

Well, here's the Tip of the Century: **When you do a body scrub, do it on dry skin.**

- You need the friction of the exfoliating particles on the dry skin cells for it to be effective. So do it in the shower, by all means, but keep the taps off. You see, if the shower is running all over your body, the buffing action is diluted, and in the case of some scrubs, the granules can dissolve before you can massage them in thoroughly. I recommend a sugar- or salt-based scrub with a lovely nourishing oil base so that it's less abrasive, has better spread and hydrates as you're exfoliating.

- Once you're done, turn on the taps and rinse it all off. Follow with a super massive giga-hydrating body butter or lotion, because *oohwee* will it penetrate beautifully now that all of those dead skin cells have racked off.

*Bonus trick!*
*One of the BEST things you can do for your skin is dry body brushing. It gets the blood and lymph flowing, exfoliates and encourages new cell growth. (And I reckon it helps smack cellulite and KP too.) Use a brush with natural bristles and, starting at the feet, move up the body, with all of the brushing movements towards the heart. It's boring, but worth it.*

239

# A TERRIFYING TALE OF CHINKLES.

Once upon a time, in a made-up land called Sydney, a young woman stumbled to the bathroom after waking up and began her usual cleanse-sunscreen-makeup face business. But something wasn't right. Something had changed...where previously the skin on her chest had been smooth, now there lived a band of renegade wrinkles. She rubbed her eyes and looked again. Yes. Yes, it was true: She had Chest Wrinkles...*Chinkles!*

The sly stepsister of crow's feet and marionette lines, chest wrinkles are the ultimate in stealth ageing. (They creep in while you sleep and, provided your skin is still supple, are only visible for a few minutes upon waking before disappearing. At least on the surface; under the skin they're settling in good and proper, waiting for the day they can hang out on your chest permanently, generously offering up your real age to anyone not fooled by your crease-free face.)

She quickly applied her face cream to the area and prayed it was just a one-off, that she'd slept funny or that her sheets had made an impression on her skin. But the next morning, same thing. Small vertical lines nestled between her sweater puppies, going up into the chest. Yes, they were faint, but *they were there*, and that was the annoying part.

She consulted some of her clever, beauty-expert friends.

'Oh yes, I always apply my face cream there, day and night. They're the secret wrinkles no one tells you about.'

'I never sleep on my side any more, that's what causes them,' said one who had a *lot* more in her cup than the protagonist did, and thus more potential of wrinkles in that area. 'I trained myself by propping rolled-up towels around my neck and head so I physically could not roll onto my side.'

'I've trained myself to sleep on my back, too,' said another big-jugged lass.

Shit sticks, the woman thought. I can't believe I've been rambling along through life not knowing that you can get wrinkles in between the cans. I mean, I knew to protect that area from the sun, and I always moisturise it, but I didn't realise there was an issue of bloody sleep wrinkles, too. So she started using her lovely rich face cream on the area every morning and night, taking special care to massage it in properly, and attempted to start sleeping on her back. *She would beat sleep's silent skin assassin!* With ease! Those chinkles could suck a doz!

But she didn't actually, because she was a sideways sleeper and her body was controlled by small invisible elves who pushed her right back onto her side each time she tried to sleep on her back.

The end.

# YOU DON'T SPRAY PERFUME ON YOUR <u>NECK</u>, DO YOU?

During the day?

Oh shit no.

Here's what you're saying to the sun when you do that:

*'How I long for a neck that is shrivelled and covered in brown spots, and for people to mistake me for a large turkey! Please burn me and create pigmentation and maybe even cause skin cancer! I would love you to! Please! OH DEAR GOD – WON'T YOU GIVE ME JUST THIS ONE SMALL FAVOUR!'*

You see, most fragrances have alcohol in them . . . and when alcohol is applied to the skin it causes photosensitivity . . . which means the skin is more sensitive to sunlight . . . which means an increased chance of both sunburn and pigmentation.

**INSTEAD:**

• Spray underneath your clothes or on your wrists. Not on your neck, not behind your ears and *definitely* not in between your cleavage.

• Spray your little index finger off at night, of course, but through the day, don't solicit sun damage for the sake of smelling like gardenia and unicorns.

# I HATE WATCHING WOMEN APPLY THEIR PERFUME.

Because they do this:

Spray perfume onto body. Rub area that has been sprayed with scent with the inside of their wrist.

**Here's the part that is right:**
Spray perfume onto body.

**Here's the part that is wrong:**
Rub sprayed area with wrist.

When you rub, you bruise all of those glorious, expensive, exquisite flowers that give the fragrance its unique scent. You violently destroy the way it's intended to slowly, gently unwind and reveal all of its depth and beauty.

So don't rub.

No more rub.

# THE BENDY BITS.

Because I sometimes yell at people who spray their perfume onto necks and behind ears during the day (sun damage and pigmentation) and on clothes (the alcohol in the juice can stain and interfere with the dyes in your pretty threads) and hair (dries it out; makes it prone to being set alight by rascals with lighters), I should probably tell you where you *should* spray your fragrance.

**BENDY BITS!**
Wrists.
Backs of the knees.
Ankles.
Inside the elbows.
Neck (if it's night-time).
Waist.

Bendy Bits tend to be warm areas and the heat from your blood flow will keep the oils in your fragrance warm enough to keep emitting fragrance. (Don't discount the knees and ankles because when your scent wears off your wrists and the thin skin behind your ears, your stilts will keep the dream alive.)

Also apply to areas like the upper back, which has little friction with other surfaces (like clothes and jewellery), which means it will dissipate over a longer time than an area that is being rubbed and the evaporation of the scent is quickened, like your collarbones or wrists.

# THREE LITTLE THINGS THAT MAKE AN OKAY SPA TREATMENT AN <u>EXCELLENT</u> SPA TREATMENT.

**1** The therapist asks if she may touch your bosom area, before diving down there to knead your chest and boobies. I'm no prude, but it can be a bit, uh, confronting to have someone leaning over you, standing behind your head, their boobs basically in your mouth, massaging your décolletage. Get the boob permission slip first, man.

**2** The therapist makes absolute certain you have no face mask remnants on your face, or mascara or eye makeup underneath your eyes before you walk out. If you do, it kind of ruins the entire 'I've just had a facial, don't I look glowy, and fresh and AMAZING?' thing that is so vital for women after having laid out cash and time to improve their face.

**3** The therapist makes sure you are lovely and warm at all times. She should keep asking, and if she doesn't, always, ALWAYS speak up and ask for another blanket or towel. Aside from a disappointing lasagne, there is nothing worse than lying down for a relaxing, peaceful body or face treatment (or being wrapped up mummy-style in a grainy body scrub) and being so cold all you can focus on is whether or not you should ask for another blanket or can the therapist turn up the heating, or perhaps remove the iceberg from the back of the room.

# ALWAYS LEAVE YOUR KNICKERS ON. ALWAYS.

Some things in beauty are obvious, like the fact that we do not eat eye cream or use nail polish on our lips. Others, though, remain confusing. Like what to do when you're given that fetching strapless terry towelling and Velcro number by a beauty therapist who is out the door before you can say, 'Enya on repeat,' and left alone in a room before a massage or body treatment. Do you strip? Do you ask for disposable grundies? Do you sit quietly and wait for the maid to come and undress you, like at home?

Thankfully, the answer is always the same. **You take off everything but your knickers**.

Now, this sounds simple, but sometimes things gets tricky. Like with Lomu Lomu massages, where they ask that you take everything off. (If they do, say you'd prefer some disposable knickers; they will *always* have some.) Or when you have opted for a relaxing twig, rock and house-paint body scrub and there is a bath or shower as part of your treatment (with the therapist involved) and they don't supply disposable knickers. And you have no spare knicks.

So I'm here to tell you, once and for all, *leave on the grundies*. You can always remove them later on if you need to, but you can NEVER get back a moment when you've none on and the therapist's hand goes just that little too high up the thigh and the awkwardness is deafening.

**The exception:** A Korean or Turkish bath house. When they say 'everything', they really do mean 'everything'. They also kind of mean, 'Or get the hell out.'

# A TRULY MULTI-PURPOSE PRODUCT: SCENTED BODY OIL.

**Something I hope you might consider after a:**

• day in the sun (lathered in sunscreen, obviously)

• lovely spray tan, or lashings of self-tan

• shower before you're about to head out for an evening of drinks/dinner/bingo

...is to mist/spritz/slather yourself in a finely scented body oil.

You'll smell better than a baby's neck. You'll glisten sexily. Your nicest body parts, like your collarbone, cleavage, shoulders and utterly ravishing legs, will be accentuated. Your tan will be emphasised.

There are a whole bunch of them out there* and many will make the need for perfume null because they smell so delicious. (Both the artificially fragranced ones and the pure, organic ones.) Some even have shimmery bronzey particles in them, which gives you a tasty bronze gleam, not unlike a Roman bust in a museum, but more film-clip babe-y, and the best ones even contain things like antioxidants to nourish as they fragrance and glisten.

*Since this book was first published I took this love for scented body oils one step further by marrying one! Also I created one called Go-To Exceptionoil and it's a goddamn multipurpose triumph and of course I'm biased but it is, and also this is my book so of course I am biased. It features ten potent and glorious skin-loving oils, and has accredited Monoi de Tahiti (from Tahiti) so it smells like a day in paradise, and will fix and soothe your skin, as well as make it smell, quite frankly, irresistable.

247

# 10 REASONS SUNBAKING IS EVIDENCE OF ARRESTED DEVELOPMENT.

Amazingly, baking your body under the single most powerful star in the universe might not be such a hot idea. I know! Next they'll be telling us smoking causes lung cancer or something.

As I am vehement, fired-up, crazy-insane about sun protection (you might be too when you learn that up to 80% of skin ageing is said to be from cumulative sun exposure, and not part of the chronological ageing process at ALL), I've put together an aggressive list of reasons why deliberate sun exposure is sheer stupidity.

1   **You can get skin cancer and die.** And when you're dead, no one gives a shit how tanned you are.

2   **The skin on your chest and arms will begin to take on the appearance of a vintage handbag,** which will make all of that botox and all of those peels kind of useless.

3   **A tan is evidence of your skin cells in trauma.** It is also a scar. The days of tans being a status symbol, and people assuming you're rich and have just been on a holiday and because you're so rich it was probably to Capri, are over. Anyone can pop over to Bali for a couple of hundo these days (or get a spray tan for $30).

4 **Ageing 'sun-kissed' babes.** These women may scrub up okay in photos, but in Real Life? Not so pretty. Ravaged by the sun and her powerful invisible ageing squadron. The result? 80 kilometres from luminous.

5 **Kate Winslet, Rachel Weisz and Cate Blanchett.** These women not only scrub up beautifully in photos, and on film, their skin belies their age even in the harshest of fluorescent lighting. They knew that wearing hats, sunscreen and covering up was going to ensure they looked 30 at 40, and 40 at 50, and 50 at 60, and probably you've figured out the pattern by now.

6 **Self- and spray-tans have come so very, very, very far.** There is, no matter how pale your skin, no reason why you cannot get a delicate sunkissed glow (or go Bahama Barbie – whatever blows your hair back) from a bottle, tube, spray gun or can of mousse.

7 **Freckles, moles, pigmentation and sunspots.** Even half an hour of incidental exposure (Incidental: When you don't account for sun exposure. Usually less than 10 minutes. Deliberate: When you know you'll be outdoors and you account for it with sunscreen etc. Make Believe: When you sit in your pretend pirate ship in a space suit and imagine you are en route to the sun) can bring on new frecks. And frecks stick around. And pigmentation is a real bitch to remove. And moles are neon signs for skin cancer.

8 **You're accelerating your ageing process.** But not just with wrinkles and fine lines on your face: actually your hands cop it the most. And you can always tell a lady's *real* age by her hands (see page 229).

9 **Halter-neck tan lines that last until May.** Nothing classier than a lovely dress being visually molested by two fat white lines. What possesses women to wear strapless dresses when they have walloping great tan lines, I don't know. (Probably the devil.)

10 **When you lie in the sun for multiple hours at a time, you are treating your body like a piece of meat being prepared for Sunday dinner** – basting it in oil and then lying in direct heat and turning occasionally. You are, quite literally, cooking yourself. I don't mean to offend, but: you are a bit of a nong.

# ACK! I'M SUNBURNED! HELP!

I'm *very* disappointed in you. Not even sure we can even still be friends. Alas, 'tis my duty to help you, even if I am secretly judging you.

**Now, just so we're all clear, here's what you've done to your skin:** Some bad shit. More specifically: sunburn is a delayed reaction to the UV radiation of the sun, specifically the UVB (B for burning) rays. When you expose your skin to the sun for too long these UV rays cause the surface blood vessels of the skin to dilate, which is what produces the redness of a sunburn. They're in agony, basically. Once the skin has been burned, the inflammation process kicks in, which includes swelling and blistering and tenderness and swearing.

**What's also happening:** The free radicals that sit quietly in your body are activated by UV exposure and turn feral and start attacking your skin cells. This is the chief cause of premature ageing. (Every time you allow your skin to be sunburned, you are speeding up your ageing process exponentially.) So get antioxidants on that skin immediately if not sooner: they neutralise the free radical damage, which means you may not need to look so old, or be quite so, um, cancerous, so soon.

**What you need to do if you are sunburned:** Initially: Swear a lot and feel stupid. Then, a cool bath or shower. Cold compress. Drink loads of water. Use a body/face lotion riddled with antioxidants (vitamins A, C and E, green tea, resveratrol, idebenone, pomegranate) immediately. Keep in mind the free radical damage from sunburn continues for 72 HOURS, so you must continue to 'antioxidant it' for at least this period. Follow up with a sun repair gel or spray on the burny areas (such as aloe vera). Take some Nurofen and some vitamin C and E capsules too. Oh, and stay out of the sun for a few days. Blisters? This counts as a second-degree burn and means you must be VIGILANT about skin cancer check ups from here on. You will likely need to dress the burn (overalls? Tuxedo? Bandages?) to prevent infection and promote healing.

**What's the rub?** As well as wrinkles and hyperpigmentation, even one bad burn can be enough to set off skin cancer cells later in life. Especially in children or skin that rarely sees the sun. So, read pages 32 and 34 again and be better at this stuff already. Okay. Thanks. Love you.

8 out of 10 women who book in a blow-dry or a spray-tan discover it's raining just as they leave the salon. If just 50% of these women went to beauty salons in areas of drought, the country's crops and livestock suffering might go down as much as 70%.

# SURE YOU'RE WEARING SUNSCREEN. BUT ARE YOU WEARING ENOUGH?

SPF only works when you use it in the way it was tested. Use not enough and you cut the SPF. Use too much and...no, that's fine, actually. Go ahead.

**In general:**

Apply sunscreen at 2 mg per cm squared.

**This means:**

Around 35ml (the equivalent of 1 teaspoon of sunscreen) should be applied to each arm, leg, front of body, back of body, and face, including neck and ears.

...based on an 'average' adult of 163 cm, 68 kg with an 82 cm waist.

Obviously if you are very tall or wide, you'll need more. These are very general guidelines and pertain to a standard, kinda thick lotion. A thinner lotion or spray* will demand more.

**Your best sunscreen ritual is:**

• Apply it 20 minutes before exposure.

• Full reapplication after water exposure (swimming, sweating, face wiping, towel-drying, dribbling), or rubbing/wiping your skin, or every two hours. Whichever comes first.

**An excellent reason to always use a very high SPF:**

Most of you probably under-apply the amount of sunscreen you need . . . which means a higher SPF could compensate for your rubbish (well it's true!) under-application.

*The jury is still out on clear sunscreen sprays. I recommend old-school lotions instead.*

# HOLY SHIT! WE'RE ALL LOW ON VITAMIN D.

We are! I read it on a Minties wrapper! It must be true! Quick, let's make sure we're on top of things.

**What is vitamin D:** A vitamin. The 'D' one. We get it from the sun.

**Why do we need it:** To maintain good health and to keep bones and muscles all strong and healthy.

**Why are we low on it:** Because we're all such GOOD kids and protecting our skin so beautifully from the sun that what is actually a crucial vitamin is being blocked.

**How to ameliorate this:** What does ameliorate mean?

**Fix. How do we fix it:** By allowing our skin to get a little sun.

**How much?** If you can give your hands and arms (around 15% of your body surface) one-third of what it would take for your skin to become faintly red daily, well that's plenty.

**For example:** In summer for fair skin, this averages around 5–9 minutes. (Getting your D-fix between 10am and 3pm in summer is *not* advised.) In winter, it might go up to around 12–15 minutes. Obviously, the amount you need varies with your skin tone, the season and the strength of the sun, so maybe do some Googling (the *Medical Journal of Australia* web site has a full list of states and seasons for Australia and NZ) and check you're getting enough for your skin/climate. Otherwise you risk rickets and osteoporosis and all manner of awful stuff.

**Bottom line:** Yes we are low on vitamin D, but in the WCS, um, scenario, I still maintain it's better to be protected from UV damage than not.

253

# YOU HAVE A MAXIMUM SUN EXPOSURE AMOUNT EACH DAY.

It's your Sun Limit and it's like having a credit card for your skin. With a *very* strictly enforced limit.

Your Sun Limit is the maximum amount of UV exposure your skin can cop per day. It's determined by things like skin type, the strength of the UV that day, your location and acclimatisation to the sun, the time of day and so on, but generally speaking you can find your Sun Limit by multiplying:

**The amount of time your skin takes to redden without sun protection**
×
**The number of SPF you use.**

So, if it usually takes you around 10 minutes to start burning in the sun, you'd times that by (SPF) 30... Which would give a maximum Sun Limit of **300 minutes**.

Once you've reached your Sun Limit, that's it, cute cat. You don't get any more. **Your skin can not take any more UV exposure**. And it proves this by penalising you with sunburn, potential skin cancers, premature ageing, sunspots and pigmentation.

Further application of product is of no use and at least 12 hours have to go by before further exposure to the sun is permitted.

Yep. The sun might be a bitch, but her accountant is even nastier.

# IS SELF-TAN:
## A) BAD
## B) TOTALLY FINE
## C) TASTY

One of the questions I am asked most is: 'Zoë, what is a crumpet? It's not toast and it's not a muffin and it's not a pikelet – what *is* it already?'

Another one, and one that is perhaps more relevant to this book is: 'Is self-tanner bad for us? Are we gonna find out it was actually carcinogenic in 15 years' time?'

In short, no. In long…

…still no. So your answer is, B. Totally fine.

The active agent in spray-tans and 99% of self- and gradual tanners is Dihydroxyacetone (DHA), which sounds moderately chemical-y and menacing and is probably what got you thinking, right? But no, DHA is simply a sugar derived from the sugarcane plant that has been used in beauty products for yeeeears. It's colourless and all it does is stain the dead surface cells on your skin, which is why you start looking brown (or, uh, orange) within a few hours.

**A slightly more nerdy explanation:** The DHA reacts with the amino acids in the dead layer of surface skin. When the amino acid and the DHA blend, they cause a reaction, the Maillard reaction. This is what causes your skin to change colour.

**I know you know this but still:** DHA doesn't protect you from the sun at ALL. So once your tan has 'bloomed', stay out of the sun, and slather on your usual sunscreen.

**I know you know this too, but still:** You're a Real Winner for choosing DHA over UVA.

**I know you don't know this:** The real reason I declined an invite to dinner last night.

# HOW TO SELF-TAN PROPERLY AT HOME.

**0** Make sure you have at least 20 minutes alone time in the bathroom. Preferably a few hours before bed.

**1** Exfoliate your skin in the shower (skin damp, taps off) using a grainy body scrub and working it in circular motions. (You may turn taps on now.) Wash it off.

**2** Dry your skin completely before applying fake tan. Put some moisturiser on dry bits like the hands, feet, knees and elbows (to prevent the tan 'grabbing') and put some Vaseline/ Papaw Ointment on your fingernails, toenails and cuticles.

**3** Get in front of a full-length mirror. Start at the feet, working up and out. Don't rub the product into the skin, just smooth it with sweeping motions over the skin so your skin can absorb it evenly. I use and highly advocate a tanning mitt. If you're using a tinted spray version, be SURE to cover the floor with a designated fake-tan towel. If you're using an invisible tanning spray, lucky you – you can even do your back.

**4** If you like a darker tan, wait 30 minutes (use your hair dryer all over your body to help dry it faster) before applying your second layer. (Or wait 24 hours if it's more of a DIY spray-tan product.)

**5** If you don't want to look darker, but you DO want to look a bit more slender/ toned, follow the tips on page 260.

**6** For spray-tan-type situations, once you're done, use a wipe or tissue to gently clean in between fingers and toes, just inside the ears and nose, and the bottoms of the feet.

**7** If you didn't use a tanning mitt, scrub your hands thoroughly (including between the fingers) and dry. (See page 259 for more tips on removing tan from hands.)

**8** If you want to maintain a glorious and believable tan, use a body POLISH, not scrub (they are much more gentle) every three days, and gradual tanner or a hydrating body lotion each morning/ night.

**9** If you *don't* want to maintain a glorious and believable tan, don't moisturise at all, especially not twice a day, and have loads and loads of jacuzzi parties and sandpaper scrubs.

## DIY SELF-TANNING PRODUCTS I LIKE AND RECOMMEND:

If I want a full, deep tan minus the spray gun... I'd use **Santorini Sun Organic Sunless Tanning Lotion**, which is a watery lotion in a deep cocoa shade, and which beautifully fakes the depth and shade of a spray tan on my medium-olive skin (I sometimes mix it with body lotion to make my own gradual tanner, *how industrious*). I also like **Ella Baché Great Tan Without Sun** lotion – it's green-based, gives a very natural colour, and is tinted so you get instant colour (phew) and can see where you're applying. (Is a bit thick and sticky at night though). **St Tropez's Self Tan Bronzing Mousse** is celebrity adored and with good reason, it gives a fantastic non-orange colour and the mousse gives good spread, making it easy to apply, and **Vita Liberata's pHenomenal 2–3 Week Tan Mousse** is sensational. It won't last *that* long, but goes on like a goddamn dream (use a tanning mitt, obviously), doesn't stink and isn't sticky. Five bronze stars.

If I want to be tanned but for it to look, y'know, natural... I would use a gel for softer, natural glow. Something like **L'Oréal Sublime Bronze Self Tanning Gel**. Or I might dilute one of my full-strength tanners with some body lotion. Or I might use **Clarins Delicious Self Tanning Cream**, because the pay-off is pretty much exactly halfway between gradual tanner and full-blown tanner.

If I want just a very subtle hint of colour... If it was, say, my wedding, or the middle of winter and a full tan might look ludicrous, I would use gradual tanner, which is a low-strength self-tanner hidden in a moisturiser, and can be selected according to your base skin tone and what level of colour you're after. I use **Eco Tan's Winter Skin**, **Palmer's Natural Bronze Body Lotion**, and **Le Tan's Daily Glow with SPF 15**.

If I needed bronzed skin immediately... At night, I'd go for something with some oomph – a matte, wash-off body-bronzing product that sprayed on instantly. **Model Co** and **Le Tan** both do them quite cheaply. (If you like shimmer, try **St Tropez's Wash Off Body**.) During the day I'd go for more of a body 'makeup' product like **Sally Hansen Airbrush Legs, DuWop's Revolotion Body Bronzing Moisturiser SPF 15**, or some fresh dirt mixed with canola oil and a sprinkle of vanilla essence. That was a joke. Don't do that.

*Tanny trick!*

*Avoid being a stenchy tanner by applying your self-tanner a few hours before bed, showering in the morning, then wearing a heavily scented body butter or oil (see page 247), which will nicely hydrate the skin and mask the lingering stink of raw potatoes.*

# HOW TO AVOID THE EAGLE.

While I very much enjoy my body being (fake) tanned and bronzed at this point in my life, I wish for my face to be bright and *non*-tanned. I even use brightening products on my face to keep it extra bright and even-toned, because I wish to have no pigmentation or brown patches there.

And it is this conflicting need to have a bright face and a tanned body that leads to what I call The Eagle: white head, brown body. So many of us love a bronzed body and a flawless, bright face, but the two together don't really work visually, unfortunately.

**So, what to do?**
Now, I can only speak for myself here, but when forced to choose one uniform shade for my body and face, I choose tanned, rather than pale all over. That might change eventually, but as I type this in my fluorescent lime bikini and white visor from the set of my latest film clip, I just can't see it.

And so, in order to cheat an all-over tanned look, I must make my pale face appear as tanned as my body: I add a little bit of tinted illuminator, bronzing gel or cream to my foundation as part of my daily makeup, then apply regular bronzer carefully, right down onto my neck and chest. (The neck is the palest part of your body; always dust some bronzer down there.)

*Bonus trick!*
*Add half body bronzer with half body oil or moisturiser and use all over skin for instant warmth when you need to show off your skin and you weren't prepared because your boyfriend forgot to tell you about this party until just now.*

# THE (ONLY) WAY TO REMOVE ORANGE STREAKS ON YOUR SKIN.

Now, I wouldn't normally stand here telling you to put household cleaning agents on your skin. (I would sit.)

But then, you wouldn't normally walk around with great neon signs around your ankles and feet and wrists, advertising that while you like to look tanned, you haven't quite mastered the art of making it look natural.

I'm not judging, sugar, my wrists are golden and my hands are white. But! There is a fix. For both of us. A MAGICAL one.

**1** Buy a Chux Magic Eraser.

**2** Rub it very gently on your orange streaks in small circles. (The white side.)

I did after reading it in a comment on some obscure blog, and now I rather like to carry on as though I thought of it. It works when lemon juice and body scrubs don't. (Like most of the time.)

*Bonus trick!*
*If your nail beds stain from fake tan, apply a layer of clear nail polish before you tan up.*

# FAKE TAN YOURSELF SOME ABS. HECK, WHY NOT!

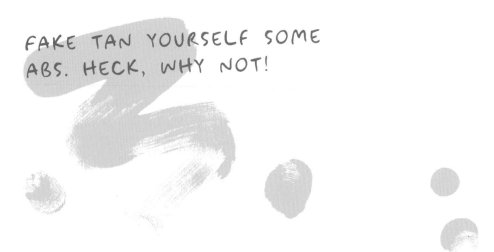

For years, professional dancers and Famous People who have to do sexy photoshoots have been tricking us into thinking they are much more toned than they are by having special tanning applications that make them look slimmer and more cut.

It's simple highlighting and contouring and shadowing, and it means you can 'hide' areas you don't love on your body, and play up (or create) 'better' parts of your body. Bloody genius. Most spray tan technicians will know what to do if you ask for a 'contouring' spray-tan (as opposed to asking for an 'edible' or 'breakdancing' one) but you can have a crack at home, too.

**First:** Using a 'spray-on' tanner, apply your usual layer of self-tan. Walk around or watch some *Family Guy* nude (NERD FANTASY ALERT!) until it's dry.

**To accentuate bits:** Choose spots where you're slim, muscular or toned (like your arms or shinbones or collarbones) and play them up by spraying on some more tanner precisely along these areas. Also spray some more over your cleavage and abs, should you have any. I certainly don't.

**To hide bits:** Apply more tanner to your less favourite areas (Thighs? Tummy? Waist? Upper arms?) using long, circular strokes, so it's kind of a soft oval shape on the skin. You do NOT want straight lines, man.

*Bonus trick!*

*After a salon spray-tan, powder on some talc into creases of knees, elbows, bum and neck area to ensure that the tanning product will not line or rub away or be affected by sweat.*

# A CLEVER TIP FOR THOSE JUICY LITTLE PITS.

If your underarms suffer from Confused Identity Syndrome, mistakenly believing they are small and efficient bathroom taps, consider this (pretty revolting) little trick:

Stick a Ladies Sanitary Pad (the real thin, new-style ones are best) on the inside underarm seam of your top or jacket. They are frightfully absorbent, and just the thing to soak up all that salty skin juice.

I know it's a little creepy, but it's a *lot* effective. And that pretty much cancels creepy out on this occasion. (Given that creepy usually wins, effective is gonna be SUCH a swell-head after this.)

If your sweating is a *real* problem, as in it's-making-you-into-a-social-dyslexic, you may want to consider botox injections in the armpits. (Or/and palms or feet.) It'll cost you around 1000 bones and will last around nine months and it will hurt a bit. But it'll make the problem go away. And sometimes that's all a lady wants, you know?

# IF YOU CAN'T TAKE THE FEET, GET OUT OF THE BATHROOM.

Obviously that is a stupid heading. But you know what I am getting at: foot beauty. Which is an equally ridiculous heading if you ask me, which you should, because I definitely know the answer.

**If your heels are dry:** Buy some Eulactol Heel Balm from the chemist, and slather it all over your heels. Put on some cotton socks and go to sleep already. It's also not a bad idea to apply some before exercise. (Making it a *good* idea.)

**If you wish to remove your grosso calluses:** For a few nights in a row, wipe some glycolic acid toner on a cotton pad (Mario Badescu does a great one you will also enjoy using on your face) over the callused area, let the skin dry, then follow with a lactic acid–based cream or lotion like DermaDrate. This will soften up your calluses and prepare them for their inevitable annihilation. Next, using a Ped Egg or equivalent, and on completely dry feet, gently 'shave off' your calluses. Undertake this ritual once a month for lovely soft feet and greatly elevated social status.

**If your feet are dry and unloved:** Find a salon that does a paraffin wax pedicure and treat yourself to one, for God's sake.

**If your feet are dry and unloved and you don't care for salons:** Make sure it's bedtime. Add Epsom salts and some lavender essential oil to a walloping big bowl and soak your feet for 10 minutes while watching something inane on TV. Dry off your feet in the bathroom, then, in the shower or bath (remember, taps off!) exfoliate them, massaging madly, with a body scrub. Rinse off, then apply an intensely nourishing cream or balm (like my very own Go-To Exceptionoil) all over the heels and feet. Rub in cuticle oil all over the nail bed and cuticles (CND Solar Oil is terrific) and slip on some cotton socks. Now get to bed, you soft-footed little scamp!

PLUG!

**If half a toenail has fallen off:** Don't for a second think you have to live with it. Go to a nail salon and have an acrylic nail attached and filed to shape. It'll take five minutes and cost five clams.

**If you are lazy like me:** Skip nail lacquer and go for gel polish on your toes. Lasts up to six weeks and won't chip. Laze-ariffic!

# THE DELICIOUS AND DIABLOLICAL ART OF PERFUME BANDITRY

The reason we ladybugs wear a 'signature scent' is so we can mischievously bully anyone who smells that perfume anywhere else at any time to think of us, and therefore we win. It is 'our' scent, the end, Amen! Suck it!

This is *especially* great when your lover smells it on another woman and thinks of you. Even if the relationship is over. *Especially* if it is over. It's just one of the many applications of perfume banditry, a wicked, wonderful little art, rare in that it is actually at its most powerful *when you're not present*.

What, you've never sprayed a pillow or a car interior with Your Fragrance so that when your lover snatched a whiff of it in your absence, he or she would immediately be forced to dwell on your loveliness? You've never chosen to wear a particular scent to a particular party knowing a particular person who particularly likes that smell will be present? Come now. Of course you have.

It's one of the most glorious, rascally pleasures of wearing fragrance.

Scent sorcery goes both ways, though, which you'll know if you've ever had the violent displeasure of smelling an ex-lover's perfume – the scent that used to make you swoon, the one you used to spray on your wrist at airports when you were forced apart – on a stranger. It's like copping an olfactory punch in the guts. But that's the price of having it work in your favour, I suppose.

Whatever. The bottom line is that perfume banditry is fun and mischievous and powerful and deliciously diabolical. Harness it as often as you can! Spray your lover's pillow! Spray a t-shirt and leave it in their car! SPRAY IT IN THEIR EYES AS THEY GAZE AT YOU LOVINGLY.

Actually, shit, shit, no, don't do that. Terrible idea. I'm so sorry.

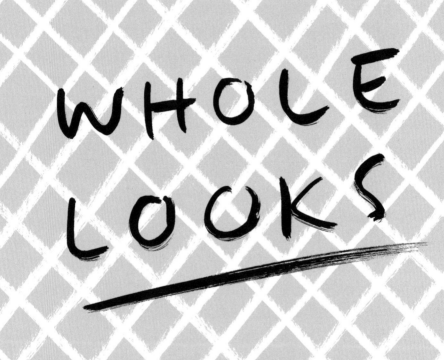

Sometimes it's not enough to just have A Lipstick Trick or A Hair Styling Tip.

Sometimes you find yourself in a situation that demands MANY BEAUTY TRICKS ALL AT ONCE, like a new job or a hangover or a lion safari.

As always, I am here to serve you.

# THE PERFECT MAKEUP FOR A MONDAY.

The combination of a face-brightening pink lipstick and bronzer is a look so fresh and so fun that if it had a hand, I would kiss it. Here's why you should wear it on a Monday.

1 It's irritatingly energetic, which is the complete opposite of how everyone at work is feeling. Amplify the effect by talking animatedly about your 'wicked boot-camp sesh' this morning as you prepare your green tea in the kitchen, not forgetting to frivolously shut the fridge with a flying jump-kick, finishing with pistol fingers and/or a playful wink.

2 As you probably/definitely won't be going out tonight, you don't need sexy-sexy eye makeup anyway. All the more reason to just focus on skin and lips.

3 The bronzer (Smashbox Bronze Lights is great, even for fair skin) will fake a healthy glow that, after a weekend of staying indoors and watching two whole seasons of *Breaking Bad*, will not be provided naturally. Just make sure you don't go too heavy: everyone knows you didn't really skip over to Maui on the weekend. Unless you live in Maui. In which case, skip to number 4.

4 It's been scientifically proven, by scientists, in proof form, that bright colours energise and stimulate the mind.

5 It distracts from your bleary, tired little eyes (speaking of which, see page 134 for how to brighten them swiftly and easily), firmly placing all emphasis on your lips. As an added bonus, bright pink lipstick makes your teeth look whiter. As an added subtraction, this means you can't have that pesto pasta today. (Try MAC Lipstick in Girl About Town or Revlon Super Lustrous in Pink Velvet.)

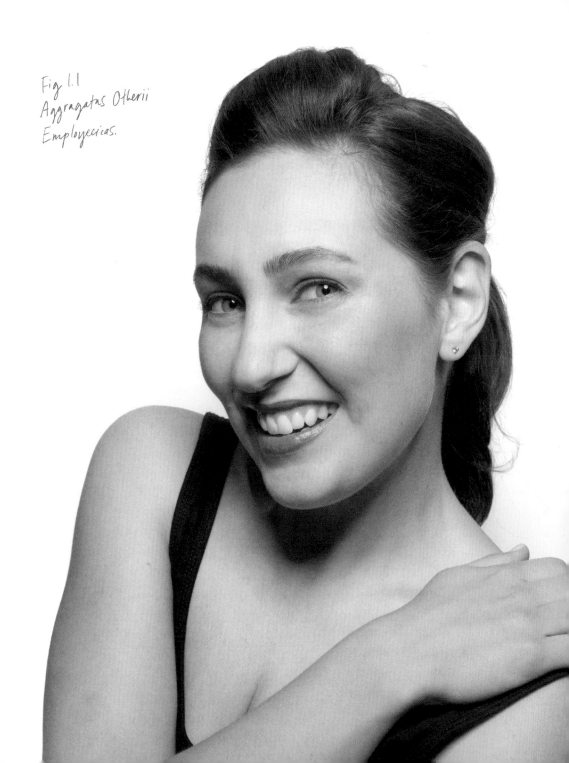

Fig 1.1
Aggragatas Otherii
Employecicas.

# OOOH, LOOK AT YOU WITH YOUR FANCY NEW JOB, FANCY JOB!

Generally speaking on your first day of a new job you want to look polished, not like you're the type who will steal stationery/petty cash/entire office desks, or the type who will be less interesting than the ink in the fax machine, or the type who will be dancing on the bar in your bra at the Christmas party (although that is kind of fun). Just *polished*.

You can crack out your wild flamingo lip tomorrow. Today, maybe we keep it simple.

*Just say some makeup inappropriately jumps onto your clothes...*
*You grab a baby wipe or makeup-removing face wipe from the super-handy pack you always have on hand, and dab the mark gently.*

**Some tips.**

- Lovely healthy cheeks – probably with a healthy flush of (non-shimmery) bronzer and blush. Or just blush.

- Natural eyes – go for a standard, inoffensive browny-taupe-based natural shadow or simple liner along the upper lash line. Then two coats of mascara.

- Grown-up lips – If you don't own a Simple Standard Nude lipstick, fill in your lips with a nudey-pink nude lip liner and then press on some lip gloss. A mouth dripping with high-shine gloss doesn't scream 'take me seriously', you know?

- Spend time the night before doing your hair, so that in the morning it doesn't misbehave and cause you to have a meltdown over something as innocuous as there being no butter left for your toast.

- Perfume – very very subtle. One spritz.

- Jewellery – probably just that big dollar-sign gold chain with the diamonds you love.

270

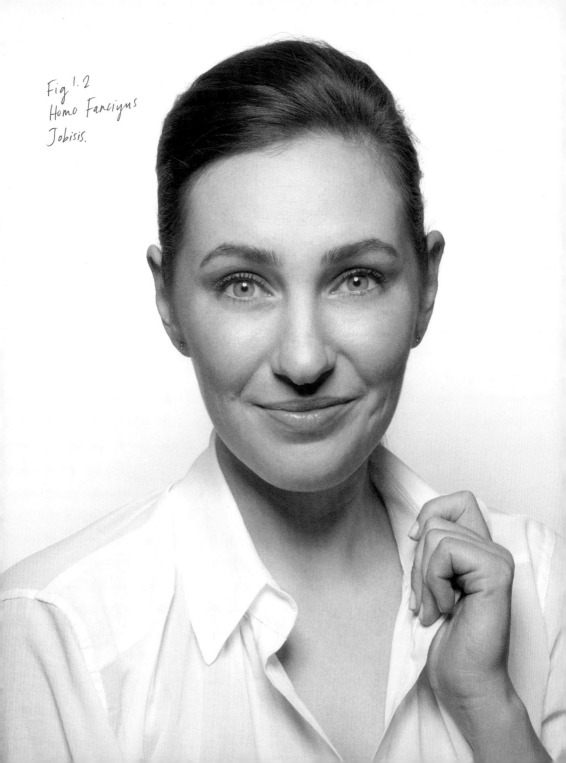

Fig 1.2
Homo Fanciyus
Jobisis.

# JUST SAY YOU WERE AFTER A CLASSIC MAKEUP LOOK.

Here would be one way to get that:

**1 Clean, semi-matte skin:**
We're after a real peaches-and-cream complexion.
Go for a medium-full coverage foundation that is not
illuminating or too shimmery. Set with loose powder.

**2 Liquid liner and upper lash mascara:**
Apply concealer and powder to your eyelids to mattify
them and cover up any veins, and then carefully apply
some liquid or gel liner across the top lash line. (See
page 110 for a cheat on this.) Apply a voluminising
mascara ONLY to the top lashes. No bottom lash
mascara. Keeps the look fresh, and the eyes more
open and . . . flirty? Fluttery? Something. Fill in and
define brows, please. (Always.)

**3 Delicious, vibrant, matte lips:**
Clean your lips of all balm. You need a clean, dry
base. Now, either apply a long-last lip liner or a
cheek/lip stain that roughly matches the lipstick you
are going to use. Then, follow with a matte lipstick.
*Matte*. It can be creamy, but not shiny. Add a whisper
of blush and you're done.No, wait, check you have
no lipstick on your teeth. All good? *Now* you're done.

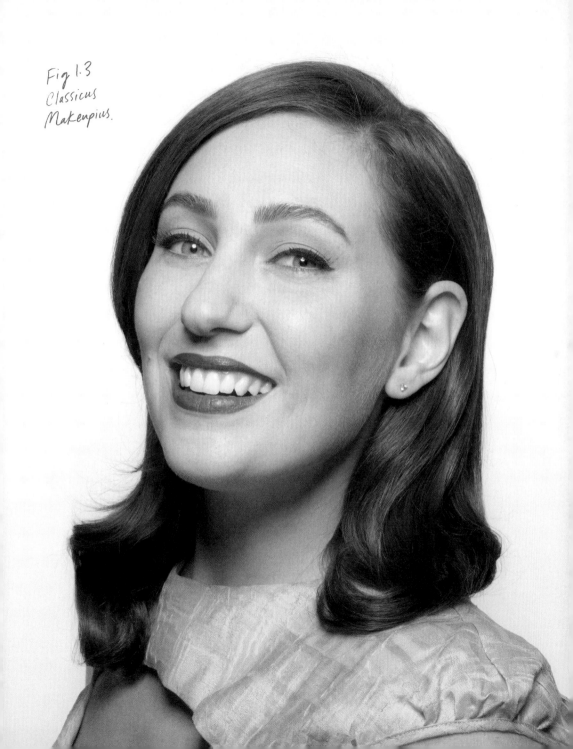

Fig 1.3
Classicus
Makeupius.

# FOUR EASY ANTI-AGEING MAKEUP CHANGES THAT MAKE A WHOPPING GREAT DIFFERENCE.

If you're glamorously gallivanting into your 50s, it's time to closely examine what you're putting on your mug every day. Because unfortunately there's a good chance it's doing you an enormous disservice.

**SIMPLE WAYS TO MAINTAIN THAT YOUTHFUL SASS.**

1 Bin those skin-drying cream foundations and stuffy face powders and immediately purchase a light-reflecting liquid foundation. That is unless you're quite happy wearing makeup that settles into your facial creases, making you appear older and far less gorgeous than is right. The difference a radiance-boosting foundation can make on a woman's face – and her perceived age – is gobsmacking. Try a skin-perfecting foundation, which offer medium to full coverage, skin-smoothing properties and hydration as well as subtle luminosity, and marvel at the difference.

**Options:** Lancôme Teint Visionnare, Perricone MD No Foundation Foundation, L'Oréal Paris NutriLift Gold Anti-Ageing Serum Foundation.

2 If you are excited with the results of your new foundation and wish to keep tearing down the anti-ageing autobahn, may I suggest you switch to a cream blush (Clarins does a lovely one that comes with a mirror and a range of extremely wearable shades) and stop using powder blush?

3 Pearly and shimmery and frosty eye shadows are very popular with mature women. Which is absurd, because they are very ageing. Instead, use matte and sheer textures, like a sheer eye shadow in a neutral shade such as soft plum, lilac or taupe. Also consider (code for 'definitely do') moving from black mascara and liner to brown – it's less harsh and far more flattering.

4 Inject colour on the lips. And the nails. There is no rule stating that as you age you must become dull. And if there *were* a rule, I would strongly advise you ignore it. Bold tones look extremely youthful. For example, coral, pink and melon lipsticks (go for a hydrating, creamy formula) look tremendously youthful, and vampy red nails never go out of style.

# HOW TO STILL LOOK GOOD WHEN YOU FEEL LIKE SHIT.

If there's one thing I know about the silly season, it's that the man it was named after, Robert Silly, sure has a lot to answer for. I mean, really Robert, *how are you meant to maintain good skin and clear eyes when you get no sleep, are stressed and eat too many spring rolls and drink too much wine!*

There *are* ways, thankfully.

**1 Tan up. Especially on the face**
This makes your eyes appear whiter immediately, and gives the illusion of activities including: yoga, green-juice drinking, meditation and sleeping. I use a full-strength self-tanner every three days, and gradual tanner each day. I do! My sheets look awesome.

As well as tanning the face, use bronzer. I can't not mention MAC Mineralize Skinfinish in Cheeky Bronze, here, which I have been using and receiving compliments on for years.

**2 Use a radiance booster under your makeup.** These contain light reflectors and illuminators as well as lovely thick moisturisers to fill in any dry lines that may have etched into your skin as a result of five Aperol Spritzes. (They're *not* primers, but will take their place in this instance.) Try: Elemis Pro-Radiance Illuminating Flash Balm or MAC Strobe Cream.

**3 Lose the matte base and heavy powders.** Go for a light-diffusing, radiance-boosting BB/CC cream or foundation, and set with translucent powder. Me? I keep a magical foundation product in my bag for touch-ups through the day and in between appointments. It's called Light Expert By Terry, and it's *unreal*.

# PREPARE YOUR SKIN AS THOUGH IT WERE IN THE SKIN OLYMPICS.

If you were to run a marathon, you wouldn't just show up on the day and expect to smash it. You would prepare. Same goes for A Big Event like your wedding, or your formal or your 30th or your graduation from fire-breathing school. You *cannot* waltz up on the day and expect your skin and hair to look as good as those birds in the magazines and on the telly unless you're prepared to put in some effort.

**THE WORK BEGINS 6–8 WEEKS OUT:**

You need daily moisturiser with sun protection and a night cream. On top of your regular skin care, incorporate a targeted serum (see page 26) and/or face oil before your night cream, and begin doing weekly facials consisting of a gentle peel (the Elemis Papaya Enzyme Peel is gorgeous) followed by a hydrating mask (like Sodashi's Brightening Marine Mineral Mask).

If you can afford it, weekly Omnilux ReVive sessions are fantastic (see page 40), moving up to two sessions in the five days leading into the event. Your skin will be an obscene shade of health.

Colour your hair a week out from the event but **no drastic haircuts.** Hair takes a while to settle in, so just get a reshape or trim, please.

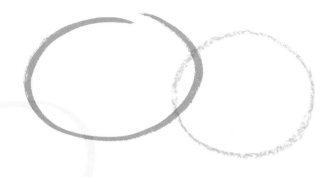

**CLOSER TO THE EVENT:**

In the interests of orange-skin avoidance, have your (light!) spray-tan (or DIY self-tan) **two nights before** (so you can scrub it off if it's too dark). Or just use a gradual tanner the day before, ideally.

If you're worried about **bloating** in that crazy-tight little dress you're going to wear, it's about Spanx, sure, but also about your diet – no salt, no booze. Try to have a green tea after each meal and drink two litres of loaded water (water with lemon or liquid chlorophyll) a day.

Have or do your **mani and pedi** the day before.

Wash your hair the night before, and have your **blow-dry or updo** done before your makeup. Splurge and pay a Makeup Counter Genius to have your makeup done. (Try Bobbi Brown or Chanel for a natural look.) It's worth it for the ease, the false lashes, how long your makeup will last and for how sensational you will look in photos. It will take up to an hour and a half. Leave enough time. And! A lot of the time, the $50 or so the makeup costs is redeemable on product. So buy a new lipstick or blush, why don't you.

Get dressed, **smile and know how incredible you look**. Also, take mints. All that dazzling visual stuff means very little if your breath smells worse than three-week-old camembert.

# ADVICE FOR A LOOOONG EVENT.

Here's some great advice that will ensure you look fresh and pretty all day at that party/wedding/the races, even when you're on your way home buying a kebab.

1 If you're having a spray-tan, have it two days before just in case it's too dark. Apply a scented body butter or lotion to hydrate the tan and mask any lingering odours.

2 A well-hydrated face followed by makeup primer is key to making your skin look good, and your makeup staying put all day (see page 68).

3 Even if you use a liquid foundation, and prefer a dewy finish, apply some translucent powder over the top to set your base.

4 Ditch the super heavy smoky eye. Rarely looks good seven hours after it was applied (and four champagnes down).

5 A classic look that's perfect for a day event: semi-matte skin, gentle blush/bronzer, winged liner on the upper lash line (and some gentle browny eyeshadow along the liner just to accentuate it), lots of lashes and a moderately colourful lipstick. You will STILL look fresh at 7pm (see page 272). And the other girls won't. Which I shouldn't point out but definitely will.

6 The more glamorous the dress, the more casual the hair. A little bit of a dishevelled bun (see page 200) is perfect for a Very Fancy dress.

7 Get your nails done. A lady who holds a glass all day must have neat, polished nails.

8 Enjoy yourself, you wild little weevil! Don't get mad if your boyfriend won't dance, or you lose an earring. In the big scheme of things, will it matter? Probably not.

# BRIDAL MAKEUP.

If, just say, you were to do your own bridal makeup (or perhaps someone else's bridal makeup), and, just say, you were not a professional makeup artist, here is a Rather Lovely look you can work with. It's natural, it's timeless, and it's designed to make you look like you, only lovelier.

**Fun fact:** Wedding makeup looks best when it's something the bride loves, is familiar with, and looks fantastic in. This is *not* a day to try something new.

**Less fun fact:** There are a lot of primers and extra steps in here, and they might seem extensive and dull, but how good your makeup looks and how long it lasts is directly proportional to the products and tools used and time put in.

### BEFORE YOU BEGIN

Squirt five drops of Rescue Remedy under your tongue, cleanse your face, and put a cloth facial mask on. (See page 24.) It'll make applying makeup a whoooole lot easier cos your skin will be all lovely and plump. No, you don't need to pick up the flowers; someone else is onto it...No, you don't need to call the photographer either...okay, know what? Just *siddown*.

### CRUCIAL PREP

Apply face cream (low SPF is better on this one occasion due to flash photography, see page 10). Wait a minute. Now apply some primer to make a perfect canvas, and hold the makeup in place all day. Do the eyelids too.

**Try:** Laura Mercier Primer (use her oil-free version if you get shine).

### APPLY FOUNDATION

Stick to what you normally use or, better still, buy a new one (trial it first the week leading up) that will give a radiant finish, but isn't shiny, and stays put. Steer clear of high SPF foundations if possible. Apply it all over the face with a foundation brush. Don't be afraid to do a few light coats.

**Try:** Giorgio Armani Fluid Sheer, Estée Lauder Double Wear Light.

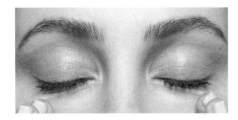

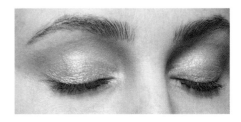

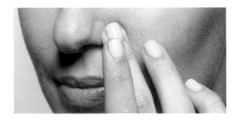

**EYES**

Apply an eye base or a primer followed by some cream eye shadow all over the eyelid as a base. Use a soft sandstone shade with a soft shimmer, and apply with a soft index finger patting motion.

**Try:** Bobbi Brown Long-Wear Cream Shadow in Stone, Shore or Bone.

Now take a shadow brush, and a neutral/brown/natural eye shadow palette, and apply a light colour (usually a soft vanilla colour) all the way from your eyelashes up to pretty much the brow bone.

**CONCEAL**

Pat in concealer under your eyes, around your nose and over blemishes. If you have an under-eye illuminator pen, apply that after the concealer (see page 87).

**Try:** MAC Studio Finish Concealer, By Terry Touch Expert Advanced.

*1.*

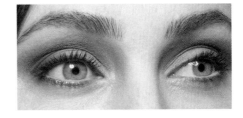

*2.*

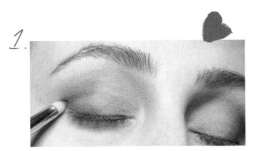

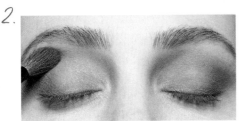

Next, using a stubby pencil brush, dab on a soft brown at the outer corner of the eye in the shape of a 'V' on its side (1), and then, using a blender brush, sweep it along and into the socket line, back and forth like a windscreen wiper, until it's all blended in (2). Keep the inside corners of your eyes and the area immediately under your brows light, to give the effect of opening up your eyes.

Take some of the darkest brown on an angled liner brush and apply it on the outer, lower area of your eyes, around two-thirds of the way along your bottom lash line. Apply a gel/cream liner with the same brush along the top lash line.

**Try:** Urban Decay Naked Eye Shadow Palette, MAC Fluidline Gel Liner in Blacktrack.

Now curl your lashes and apply some lengthening, volumising *waterproof* mascara (like CoverGirl LashBlast Volume Waterproof Mascara). High risk of tears, y'see.

And finally, define and fill in your brows with brow powder, and set in place with brow gel. Do NOT skip this step, you rascal. (See page 135 as to why.)

**Try:** Laura Mercier Brow Powder Duo, Benefit Gimme Brow.

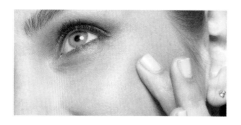

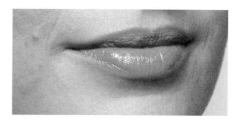

## CHEEKS

Apply a natural pink blush on the apples of your cheeks with a blush brush (see page 80), or your finger if it's a cream blush, and skim the top of your cheekbones with subtle, non-shimmery highlighter.

**Try:** MAC Powder Blush in Springsheen; Hourglass Ambient Lighting Palette.

## POWDER

Gently dust some translucent powder over the T-zone (or the whole face if you get shiny) for staying power.

**Try:** Laura Mercier Translucent Loose Setting Powder.

## LIPS

Line the lips with a nude-toned, long-last liquid lipstick or liner. Let it set, then paint on an almond or sweet dusky-pink lipstick with a lip brush. Gloss will slip off and doesn't come up that great in photos, but take some with you for touch-ups later on.

**Try:** CoverGirl Outlast All-Day Lipcolor in Always Rosy, Clinique Colour Surge Butter Shine Lipstick in Delovely.

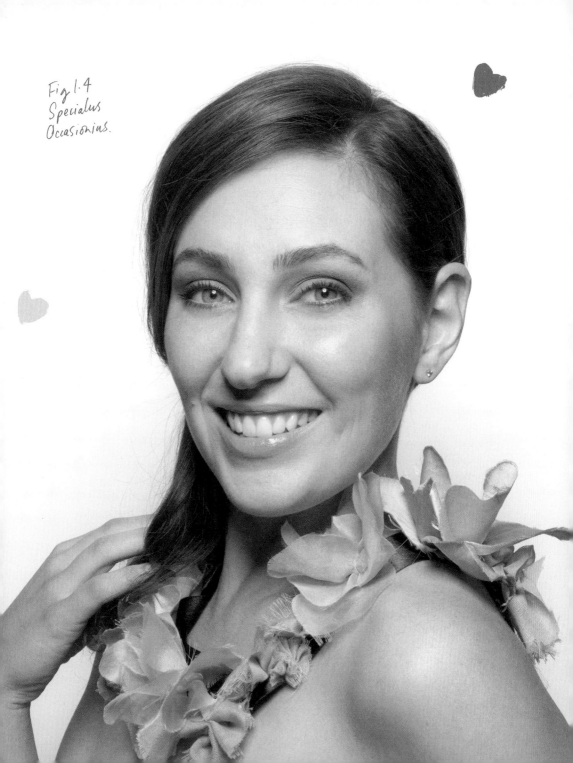

Fig 1.4
Specialus
Occasionius.

# HOW DO YOU DO YOUR FACE WHEN YOU'RE HUNGOVER?

Is it the same as when you are not hungover? Yes? Great! And by great I mean WRONG.

Provided you are over the age of 25, you just cannot use the same skin care and makeup the morning after 14 million drinks. It will not work. You need special assistance. Special products. Allow me to list some of them for you. (I apologise to those who have oily skin – these tips may not suit you because they are deliberately intended to create sheen, and if you have oily skin, this is the very thing you avoid. But! Remember: Even oily skin can be very dehydrated.)

- Drink three large glasses of water. Powerade too, if available. If not, make it available.

- Shower. (Try to stand during this if possible.)

- Exfoliate face so that all face creams have a better chance of penetrating skin.

- Use eye makeup remover on kohl remnants. Quite extensively.

- Apply eye drops to clear up redness.

- Pop on a hydrating face mask for 5–10 minutes.

- Apply a hydrating serum if possible, or massage in some face oil.

- Apply a thick face cream/daily moisturiser with SPF. Your usual face cream will not cut it today because your skin is going to be so dry. This is because selfish organs like the brain and liver are using up all the available water in your system after you decimated your hydration levels with all those margaritas.

- Apply primer. This is crucial because your skin will be so thirsty it will eat all your makeup no matter how much you apply. Primer is your best chance of keeping it in place.

- Apply a dewy BB/CC cream, or foundation. Please do not use powder or matte foundations if possible, mineral notwithstanding. The idea is to reflect light, to make your face glow. Use blotting paper if you're worried about shine.

- Use bronzer. MAN, will this make a difference – your face will look warmer; less dead-like (see page 72).

- Use cream blush in a bright shade on the apples of your cheeks. This will 'lift' your face. Give you some health.

- Use some flesh-toned liner on the inner rim of the eyes (see page 108). A little black liner on the outer corners of the top lash line. Curl lashes. Lots of mascara.

- Drink some more water.

- Use a lovely juicy gloss that has a pop of bright colour. Tremendously fresh.

- Apply some lovely perfume so you at least smell good even if you still – despite all of the incredible trickery just detailed – look like shit.

- Head to the nearest cafe for a banana smoothie (potassium), a bacon sandwich (grease), and a quadruple-shot espresso (personality).

# LOOK GOOD AFTER A LUNCHTIME WORKOUT.

If you're anything like me (four legs, bushy tail, penchant for worms), you're always running or at the gym on your lunchbreak, just pumping iron and lifting weights and doing jazzercise and elliptical-ing away. But what of the post-gym bit, where you gotta look presentable when you shimmy back to the office/hotdog stand, but your face is red and you look a cute, fit mess? If only there were a book right in front of you that could assist...

- It's best to remove makeup *before* working out (use face wipes instead of cleanser – faster! easier!) to avoid breakouts, but I keep my eye makeup on to speed things up at the other end.

- Shower, as cold as you can to get that core temp down.

- If, like mine, your face goes lobster red after exercising, and stays that way for 1000 hours, then you need to both calm the skin and conceal the blazing red. Apply a calming moisturiser (an anti-redness one, if possible) to calm the redness and inflammation, because if you are prone to redness, heat plus sweat will not be your friend.

- If you are heading outdoors again, apply sunscreen. Remember: Chemical sunscreen goes onto clean skin; physical sunscreen goes on after face creams, etc., just before makeup. See page 32 for a super fun reminder! #LOL #sunfun #factsarecool # 😄

- You *might* want to conceal redness with a green-tinted primer or colour correcting product here (so your foundation has less heavy lifting to do).

**Options include:** L'Oréal Paris Studio Secrets Color Correcting Primer or Make Up For Ever HD Microperfecting Primer (good for dry, flaky skin).

- Now apply foundation or a CC cream (CC stands for colour corrective, making them ideal in this situation) that will help disguise redness and give medium coverage.

  **Try:** La Roche-Posay's Rosaliac CC Crème or Smashbox Camera Ready CC Cream.

- Conceal around the nose, below the eyes and the eyelids, which are bound to be redder than usual from all those blood vessels beaming with happy, oxygenated, exercisey blood.

- No blush. Zero blush.

- If you have no eye makeup on, do two coats of mascara. As Plato once said, 'When the face is red and the hair is grimy, make sure your lashes are coated and shiny.'

- Nude gloss is best – wearing a brightly coloured lipstick with a flushed face will only accentuate redness. Wait till your skin has calmed down, then pop colour back on.

- Hair? Go to page 216 please.

- Now spray on some perfume, grab your stinky gym bag and get back to work, you fit, beautiful son of a bitch.

# THE MAGIC OF DAY-BEFORESIES.

When I need to look breathtaking for an event, I wear a full-body Gigi Hadid mask. If that's in the wash and I have to go as myself, I start prep the Day Before. This allows things to settle in and relax a little.

Think of the day after an event when your hair has body but is soft and sexy, and your tan is perfect, and you have some eyeliner still hanging around your eyes making them seductive and rock and roll. Like that. Also, it gives you time and room for error, should there be any (orange wrists, boofy blow-dries, breakouts).

**HAIR**

Hair doesn't behave when it's freshly washed. It's slippery, fluffy and frizzy. So, wash it the night before your event and enjoy the pliability of second-day hair instead. More specifically, wash then apply mousse or a styling balm all over, and blow dry it so that it's dry and smoothish. The next morning, spray heat protectant all over and style away, with your hair dryer, tongs or styler. You will have a good base and your style – be it out or up – will hold better and for longer. You can even have your salon blow-dry the day before if your hair, like mine, looks too perfect, too bouncy, too...not me, when it's freshly done and glistening with hairspray. But the next morning it has dropped and is real good.

**TAN**

Don't self-tan or have a spray on the day, even though there are two-hour spray tans available. The day before is better: it means you will have had a chance to wash off the tint, and the stank will be gone. On the day, have a lukewarm shower then apply a thick, fragranced body lotion, butter or balm to lock the tan in and mask any stench. If there are areas of build up around the 'bends' – elbows, knees, ankles or wrists – use a body scrub and lemon juice to dilute. (If it's still too dark, soak in the tub for halfa. Or go to page 256.)

## SKIN

Facials are wonderful when you want your skin to RADIATE, but don't expect to look good the day of: you'll be red, blotchy, roughed up and sticky, and have small pieces of mask on your jawline. The next day, though...[sleazy wolf whistle]. The skin will be plump and glowing, your eyes will be bright and clear, and your makeup will look extraordinary.

If you're having a peel or any kind of microdermabrasion, then do it 5–7 days before. You don't want to risk flaky or peeling skin.

**The exception:** at-home mini-facials before an event. Exfoliate then do a quick 10-minute hydrating or brightening mask.

## NAILS

These are fine to get on the day, but you can get them done easily and quickly a day/night or two before with no consequences. Plus, sometimes nails can look a bit raw and ouchy right after a mani, especially if you choose a dark colour and a shitty manicurist brutalises your cuticles.

**Fun fact:** if you got gels and hate the colour because it makes your hands look like Aunty Edna in her casket (poor dear, she was such a beast on the tennis court), paint over them with a coat of regular nail polish. It can be removed again with polish remover and your gels will remain perfect.

## MAKEUP

No no no, definitely do this on the day, you banana.

# FIVE
## ways to make your look last.

You know how when you build a house, you have to create a frame for the house, and drill steel poles into the ground to anchor the house safely, and sprinkle dragon-wing dust on the site so that you are protected from trolls? Of course you do! This crucial groundwork and vital scaffolding ensures a strong foundation for your house so that it is durable and it lasts. Cosmetics are no different. Albeit with less concrete.

Everything you do to your skin, body, face and hair needs to be done with proper preparation or it will fall apart as soon as it's tested by the elements (heat, humidity, wind, dryness), or the clock, or your penchant for high-energy, vodka-fuelled jazz ballet when you go out on a Friday night.

## 1.

**Face.** Apply primer on top of your skin care, followed by your base and concealer. Now the colour stuff – brows, blush, bronzer, eye shadow, etc. Then, with a large, fluffy brush, lightly dust your entire face with loose powder, or mineral loose foundation, to set it all in place for the day. (If you have oilier skin, you might prefer pressed powder.)

## 2.

**Body.** Midway through your shower, turn off the taps. Fully exfoliate your body with a body scrub (make your own with two parts brown sugar, one part olive or coconut oil, and mix together), going in circular motions to get rid of dead skin. Turn on the shower and rinse. Dry off thoroughly, wait a few minutes, then apply self-tanner all over with a tanning mitt. Moisturise am and pm, and use a gentle body polish in the shower every 2–3 day before applying gradual tanner.

## 3.

**Lips.** Apply lip balm before doing the rest of your makeup. When it's lip time, gently, with tiny strokes, fill in your lips with either a lip liner that matches your lipstick, or – better yet – a multipurpose nude liner, which will work with every lipstick, and in fact will make their pigment seem truer. What a gas! (I like Stila Glaze in Mocha, MAC Lip Pencil in Spice and Rimmel Lasting Finish 1000 Kisses in Wild Clover.) Next, paint on your lipstick with a lip brush. Kiss a tissue to blot (no Frenching, you sicko) and then paint another layer on.

## 4.

**Nails.** Remove old polish, file and buff, push down your cuticles and remove all traces of hand creams and oils by running a damp cloth over each nail. Apply base coat to each nail and then wait a minute. Apply your first layer of colour, starting on the sides of each nail and then filling in the middle. On the second coat, finish each nail with a tiny swipe across the actual edge/top/tip of the nail, to seal the colour. Wait a minute, then apply topcoat. Refresh your topcoat every second day for TURBO longevity. I like Orly Glosser High Shine Topcoat, and also Sally Hansen Mega Shine, which dries quick and is shiny and thick enough to mask the inevitable nudges and scrapes I acquire 22 minutes after a manicure.

## 5.

**Mop.** Apply mousse or root lifter or texture spray to freshly washed hair: anything that will create some hold and grip and body. Now blow dry the hair off because heat makes products work, and damp hair gets greasy real quick. If you launch into a full-scale salon-style blow-dry, the bounce and thickness and smoothness will delight. If you apply some heat protectant spray and use your styler or curling wand for waves, they will hold shape and look better for days. Bring in your *dry* styling products (volume powder, dry shampoo, hairspray, pomades, shine sprays, etc) once the hair is styled for finishing touches.

# Q + A

You know what they say: There's no such thing as a dumb question, but there IS such a thing as an idiotic question.

I ignore 'them', though, they're mean. I reckon any question is a good question. Even ones where the answer is obvious, like: 'Should I buy a copy of Amazinger Face for each of my friends, or two copies?' (Two.)

Anyway. Following are some useful questions I've been asked. Whether the answers are useful remains to be seen, but let's all pretend they are and pour some rosé already.

# Q: WHAT ARE PARABENS AND WHY IS EVERYONE SO TERRIFIED OF THEM?

Parabens are a group of chemicals used as preservatives to stop bacteria growing in food, cosmetics and therapeutic products. You'll see them in the ingredients list under names like methylparaben, ethylparaben, propylparaben, butylparaben and isobutylparaben. Some fantastic options in there for those looking for a truly unique baby name.

When a study in 2004 revealed parabens were a contributing factor to breast cancer, people FUH-REAKED. However, it's since been shown that there's no conclusive evidence to suggest using products containing parabens is directly linked to the development of cancer. Also, the research linking them to cancerous cells is unsatisfying, as it didn't compare results with paraben levels in non-cancerous cells, i.e., there was no control group. All of that said, as with all things we consume and slather on our skin, more investigation is justified and necessary.*

Australia is lucky to have one of the strictest cosmetic regulatory systems in the world (the Therapeutic Goods Administration, or TGA) and at the time of print, the TGA maintains there's not enough evidence to prove parabens are hazardous, especially in small doses in cosmetics.

However. If you're prone to allergies, sensitivity or irritation, you may be reacting to parabens, in which case it's best to avoid them, and other things that can cause flare-ups, like fragrances and hearing the same Taylor Swift song too often. Thankfully, as collective awareness of 'nasties' grows, there are plenty of paraben-free skin care ranges around (WARNING!! PLUG!!!) including my own, Go-To, so you can easily live a paraben-free life.

Other stars in the skin care nasties line up:

**PEGs (polyethylene glycol):** A mix of compounds and polymers used as emulsifiers or emollients, or to keep ingredients stable. PEGs themselves aren't bad guys, but since they enhance absorption of other ingredients, they could be fast-tracking chemical undesirables into your skin.

**Sodium lauryl sulfate/sodium laureth sulfate (SLS and SLES):** These make things foamy, are absorbed into the body and are known to be skin, lung and eye irritants. Plus, they interact and merge with other chemicals to form nitrosamines, most of which are carcinogenic. What jerks.

**Petroleum and mineral oils:** Petroleum derivatives that coat the skin and stop it from breathing, absorbing and excreting. They do nothing to nourish the skin, they just sit on top.

*I am a stunning tap dancer and a writer, but no scientist. There's a lot of hysteria and research to wade through regarding parabens, which is the reason I refer (and ultimately, defer) to the TGA – they are the regulatory body put in place to protect consumers/cuties like us.

# Q: DO I NEED TO USE TONER? REALLY?

 **A:**

Toners get a bad wrap because they seem superfluous and dated, but they are neither. They are useful and can dramatically transform very dry or very oily skin! Any skin, in fact!

**Toners can do all this stuff:**
- Ensure thorough removal of any makeup, primer and sunscreen your cleanser missed.
- Rebalance oil levels and reduce oil production.
- Restore pH levels.
- Clear out clogged pores (which lead to breakouts) and minimise their appearance.
- Help with hyperpigmentation, wrinkles, acne, etc.
- Deeply hydrate.
- Calm and soothe red/irritated skin.
- Allow OPTIMAL serum and moisturiser absorption.
- Give makeup a better chance of lasting and sitting better on the skin.
- Reverse park without using any mirrors.

As well as thrilling modern formulas with exciting new benefits, some toners even come in mists that take less time to use than it takes to swoon over Tom Hardy, making them excellent for busy/lazy peanuts like you and me.

**Oily skin/breakouts:** Go astringent, as in a more 'traditional' toner. They will clean out and tighten pores to stop breakouts and excess oil production. Mario Badescu's Special Cucumber Lotion is well recommended.

**Combination skin:** You need something balancing, to keep the oil in check, add moisture to dry patches, and gently clean your skin. Look for the words 'balancing' and 'combination' on the bottle. Origins makes a popular one called United State Balancing Tonic.

**Hyperpigmentation:** Look for words like 'whitening' and 'brightening' and be sure to use sunscreen each day as this toner may utilise AHAs, and as AHAs are an exfoliant, they leave your skin more vulnerable to UV damage.

**Mature skin:** Go for one with AHAs to help gently resurface the skin and help skin cell renewal, like Alpha-H's Liquid Gold.

**Dry skin:** Skip alcohol (topically, anyway) and acids for antioxidants. One option is Aesop's Parsley Seed Anti-Oxidant Facial Toner.

**Normal skin needing hydrating and clarifying benefits:** You don't need the astringent stuff or actives. SK-II's Facial Treatment Essence is gorgeous.

**Sensitive skin:** Go as pure as possible to avoid any irritation and help calm the skin. I love the Sodashi Rejuvenating Face Mist.

## Q: HOW DO I GET RID OF THESE RIDICULOUS LARGE PORES?

**A:**

You cannot get rid of your big pores, or change their size. What you CAN do, though, is ride bikes and eat ice cream, so it all comes out in the wash.

Sorry, that was a truly pore response. I can do better. (*Zzzzing!*)

Now. While you can't change your pore size (it's genetic) or stop them overproducing oil, or creating pimples or blackheads, you *can* diminish their appearance and sheen using a skilful artillery of pore-minimising products, designed by people who understand that while bigger, oilier pores generally mean your skin will age more slowly and wrinkle less (good thing), they don't always look that great (bad thing).

**Skin care**

- Cleanse thoroughly, you cute little pig: the key to keeping pores in check is ensuring they're clean. The dirtier they are, the more visible they become. Use something gentle, so as to really clean but not over stimulate sebum production. Obviously I am going to recommend my own Go-To Properly Clean here. Duh.

- Exfoliate at least 2–3 times a week. Too much exfoliation can aggravate the pores and make them produce *more* oil. Adorable! Something with AHAs or BHAs (salicylic acid) or a combo of both is terrific.

- After cleansing, use toner. This 'closes' the pores and tightens them without drying them out (and if it *is* drying them out, switch products). Lancôme Tonique Pure Focus is popular, as is Bioré's Triple Action Toner.

- Use a serum targeted to pore (size/ visibility) reduction.

- Moisturise and use sun protection; UV damage further enlarges pores.

- A weekly mask to draw out impurities is necessary. Something like the much lauded SkinCeuticals Clarifying Clay Masque is perfect since it uses clay. Clay is the way. *Clay is the way.*

**Makeup**

- Not yet! First apply a pore-reducing primer to do all the heavy lifting, effectively 'sealing' up your pores to create a lovely, smooth canvas for your foundation. There are loads around but people go especially nuts for Benefit's POREfessional and Smashbox Photo Finish Targeted Pore & Line Primer.

**Now makeup**

- Use mattifying or 'pore-minimising' foundation to conceal the appearance of larger pores and keep oil under control. Revlon Colorstay Makeup, Maybelline Dream Matte Mousse and bareMinerals Matte SPF 15 Foundation all get a good wrap.

- Keep blotting papers (or a powder compact) on hand for touch-ups.

I know that sounds like a lot of work, but that's only because it is. Can't be arsed? *At least* do the exfoliating and toning, and use a primer.

# Q: HEY ZO, WHAT ARE YOUR THOUGHTS ON...

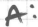

### Colonics?
A wonderful, albeit slightly confronting and giggly way to boost a detox, and a terrific idea before and after long-haul flights, or if you have been too much of a party cat lately, or if you're feeling unhealthy and sluggish and looking to kick your own arse (er, literally) into a healthier, cleaner gear. I go for the 'closed' method. For obvious reasons.

### Invisalign?
An alternative to braces for teeth straightening. As a chronic night-time grinder with slightly overlapping front teeth, this was the perfect solution for me. Mostly to stop the grinding, which was causing all kinds of mischief in my gums and playing havoc with my teeth line, but if the by-product happened to be straight teeth, well, I was willing to valiantly suck it up. I wore the tight, clear trays and the little 'teeth horns' for six months, and now just wear regular trays at night. Highly recommend!

### Fraxel DUAL?
I tried the Fraxel DUAL, a laser that is designed to boost the skin's collagen, which stimulates the growth of new skin cells to enable skin healing and promote skin renewal, and used most commonly for dark spot removal. I was trying to clear some *minor* hyperpigmentation, and regret doing this. As well as the standard swelling and peeling, I had

(FOUR!) cold sores come up, and the result complexion-wise was barely noticeable. Then soon after, I realised my pigmentation was worse. I put this down to the trauma and heat of the treatment causing more inflammation, old pigmentation coming up to the surface, and new pigmentation appearing on the new, fresh, vulnerable skin. I was advised to have another round or two but politely declined. This may have been helpful, but I was too battle-scarred. So, if you're considering Fraxel or similar for hyperpigmentation, be cautious: there are different kinds of hyperpigmentation, and inflammation creates different reactions from person to person.

**Hypoxi?**
A range of gentle workout machines that target stubborn fat deposits on the bum, tummy and thighs, Hypoxi suits all body types and ages, especially 'fat-skinnies' who do everything right in the gym and diet but can't tone up those lady jiggles. I love Hypoxi. After a 12-session program, I see results: many centimetres lost around my lower tum, bum and thighs, incredibly taut skin tone, some weight loss, and even my cellulite buggers off. It was especially great for toning up when I couldn't do any exercise after pelvic/hip issues post-birth.

**Wearing a suit made of ice?**
Meh. It wasn't quite as warm as I would have liked.

# Q: HOW DO I REMOVE MASCARA PROPERLY?

Depends where you put it. If it's on your sofa, try some Jif. If it's on your eyelashes, then it's a little more involved.

**Regular mascara?**

Use a dual-phase oil and water remover (like Lancôme Bi Facil) for quick and very efficient results (but a no-no with lash extensions). These are good if you wear a lot of liner and shadow with your mascara. Or just stick to a regular, water-based eye makeup remover. Be sure to hold the cotton pad over the closed eye, then wipe down the lashes (not horizontally – very wrinkle-causey). Better still, use eye makeup pads (see page 115).

**Waterproof mascara?**

Use cleansing oil, which is moisturising, gentle and ace for removing makeup and dirt without disrupting your skin's barrier. Cleansing oils emulsify once you add water and massage them onto (dry) skin, then glide off as you rinse, so there's no need to cleanse afterwards, though you can and it's fine. And yes, even oily skin can (should!) use them – the oil takes away not only makeup and grime, but also excess sebum. If you're a heavy makeup

(especially long-last or waterproof), primer or sunscreen user, cleansing oil is for you. I like shu uemura Cleansing Oil and Dermalogica's PreCleanse.

**Tubular mascara?**

Tubular mascara is applied like regular mascara, but quietly and invisibly creates little tubes around each lash. This means it won't smudge or fall off, it just stays PUT, hugging each lash like a lover. Sweat, cry, be in the tropics; it won't budge. But the REAL bonus is that no makeup remover or cleanser is required to remove tube mascara – just warm water to soften the tubes, and your thumb and forefinger to gently slide the 'tubes' down and off the lashes. I'm a total tubular tragic.

**Lash extensions?**

If you use mascara on your lash extensions, avoid waterproof and tubular mascara and deffo AVOID OIL-BASED REMOVERS. Use regular mascara and remove very gently with a water-based remover, or, if you are good at magic, just remove it quickly using a rudimentary spell.

# Q: WHAT ARE BB CREAMS AND CC CREAMS AND ZZ CREAMS?

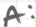 A:

One thing I am asked a lot is, What are BB and CC creams, will they change my life and do they taste any good when dipped in tzatziki? Ignoring the idiotic last bit, here is my answer: Generally speaking, BB and CC creams are souped-up tinted moisturisers.

**BB creams** vary in their offerings and finishes, but usually are a blend of:

• Moisturisation

• Light sun protection

• Primers or skin-perfecting ingredients

• Sheer coverage

• Skin care ingredients (antioxidants, etc.)

…making them great for the time-poor or lo-fi, those who don't like to wear makeup, or those who have good skin and don't need much coverage.

BUT. I'd be very cautious relying on them to do all things. For one, the amount of moisturisation and the amount of sunscreen in many BBs is simply not enough, so you need a dedicated SPF 30 moisturiser underneath. I reckon a single product can do two, maybe three things well: any more than that and *all* its benefits are diluted.

**CC creams** refer to colour correction, the idea being they conceal (and treat) dark spots/uneven skin tone (hyperpigmentation), redness and sallowness while maintaining a healthy, luminous finish. They often contain whitening/brightening ingredients as well as moisturiser, plus sunscreen and light-diffusing particles, but they're closer to foundation in coverage. I love CC creams. They bridge the gap between BBs and foundation perfectly, and only when I need Really Lovely Proper Makeup do I use foundation instead of a CC.

**ZZ creams** don't exist. Sorry.

# Q: HOW DO I FIX THIS GODDAMN HYPERPIGMENTATION?

 **A:**

Hyperpigmentation (melasma, sun spots, age spots, dark spots, brown marks and the 'mask of pregnancy' a.k.a. chloasma) is so common among Australian women that my statistics calculator broke when I asked it for percentages.

It's real easy to get, just ask your face after a few days on a beach. This is because hyperpigmentation is (most often) caused by UV exposure. UV stimulates the pigment cells (melanocytes) in our epidermis to start making melanin. This is what causes suntans (*sooo* '80s) but also hyperpigmentation.

There is **epidermal** pigmentation, which is surface-level and generally sun-related and treated easily with topical brightening products; and there is **dermal** pigmentation, which sits lower in the skin, and which requires more invasive treatments.

**Other causes:**

• Heat can trigger hyperpigmentation. This is so incredibly shit because even if you are vigilant about your skin care and sun protection and hat and sunnies, thermal heat encourages melanocytes to produce melanin! Damnit!

• Hormonal hyperpigmentation looks like UV hyperpigmentation, but has a bitchier attitude and eats more Tim Tams. It's generally caused by external hormones (the pill) or internal hormones (pregnancy) and is further exacerbated by sun.

• Know how after pimple-picking you get that red-browny scar that won't leave, no matter how much rosehip or vitamin E oil you use on it? That's because it's not a scar, it's post-inflammatory hyperpigmentation, which comes about after trauma to the skin. It can also happen after needles, injections, burns – any inflammation.

Aside from the daily annoyance of brown spots, uneven skin tone is visually FAR more ageing than wrinkles. It is! Bright, even-toned skin still looks youthful and luminous even when it is lined and creased.

There are SIX BILLION products and treatments for hyperpigmentation, and I'd know cos I have tried 102% of them. The best advice I have is to seek a proper skin consultation to determine what kind of pigmentation you have, then work out the most appropriate course of treatment/action/product usage for you. Don't waste time/money/effort and potential great skin by guessing.

**The Rules of Hyperpigmentation Club:**

**1** Be patient! It's a maddening, time-consuming process. Most products will take at least 4–6 weeks until results can be seen, and in-salon treatments may take three times that.

**2** Be diligent! No point buying a stack of products and treatments if you neglect to wear a physical sunscreen every single day, and cover your face thoroughly outdoors. The brown spots are lingering under the surface, like a creep, waiting for a chance to come back. Don't let them.

**3** Something about not talking about Hyperpigmentation Club.

**HOW TO PREVENT AND TREAT HYPERPIGMENTATION:**

· Use a **pigment blocker/inhibitor** each morning and night on clean skin to prevent pigmentation triggering in the first place, which means less time treating it. There are tyrosinase inhibitors (e.g: kojic acid, mulberry extract) that work to block the enzyme tyrosinase which is needed to make melanin. There are also PAR-2 inhibitors, like soy and niacinamide, which can result in reduced melanosomal transfer and distribution, leading to a lightening of skin pigmentation. Options include: CosMedix Simply Brilliant, or Aspect Pigment Punch.

· **Chemical exfoliation** in the form of AHAs or BHAs can remove the cells with pigment, or the 'expression' stage of pigmentation, by helping the skin to shed old cells and allow pigmentation to break down and move to the surface where it's slowly eliminated, leaving a more even-toned complexion. (Ideally.) Look for ingredients like glycolic acid, lactic acid, citric acid and salicylic acid, or even retinol. Your exfoliation can be in the form of a cleanser, toner, serum or moisturiser, or a dedicated exfoliant. Less is more here: overusing aggressive actives leads to inflammation, which leads to more hyperpigmentation. Oh, the fun! I like Alpha-H's Liquid Gold, Ultraceuticals' Even Skintone Serum and SkinMedica Lytera. Look for words like 'whitening' and 'brightening' and 'even-tone'.

- **Wear a broad-spectrum (UVA and UVB) physical sunscreen** (one with zinc oxide or titanium dioxide) on top of your pigment blocker every single day. (See page 32.) This is crucial to stop UV damage, but also because when using AHAs or BHAs you MUST wear sunscreen every day. Some ingredients in chemical sunscreens can actually trigger hyperpigmentation, so I steer clear. And no, the sunscreen in your BB cream is not enough, before you ask. You need dedicated sun protection, especially if you're battling hormonal pigmentation.

- Finally, use as many **anti-inflammatory ingredients and antioxidants** in your face creams and oils and serums as possible: they're helpful for overall skin health but especially great at stopping free radicals from causing havoc. (I made face oil that is SUPER anti-inflammatory and filthy with

antioxidants called Go-To Face Hero for this very reason.) Vitamin A is also recommended: it's one of the only ingredients dermatologists all agree can change and correct the skin (due to its ability to correct damaged DNA), and as it helps channel damaged cells to the surface of the skin, it speeds up the lightening process. Only use vitamin A under the supervision of a trained skin care expert. A trained monkey will not suffice.

With regards to **professional treatments such as lasers, Fraxel, IPL**, etc., I urge caution. These are inflammatory procedures, capable of causing trauma and post-inflammation pigmentation... It's a vicious, bitchy cycle. I had Fraxel a few years ago and it made it worse: old pigment came through and new pigment popped up while my skin was vulnerable. Plus, you have to basically live as a vampire if you go down the laser route cos even a few hours in the sun can undo months of skin-brightening work. I know! I know. FFS.

I stick to inflammation-free treatments like strong lactic peels, (occasionally) combined with microdermabrasion and vitamin C infusions to combat my (epidermal, i.e., top layer) pigmentation. And I keep up the at-home stuff as detailed above. And I wear hats. And carry around a mobile fridge to keep me cool.

# Q: I'M A BROKE STUDENT, WHAT SKIN CARE DO I NEED?

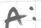 **A:**

Ahhh, I remember this world. It's riddled with heavy, expensive university textbooks, well-priced beers, triple-shot coffees, cheap movie tickets, and not nearly as much yachting and couture as one would like.

Luckily, provided your skin is in Fairly Good Shape (that is, no full-blown acne or sensitivity/redness, etc.), you can get away with a pretty simple and cost-effective routine.

**It should include:**

A simple, gentle cleanser that also removes makeup. Micellar cleansing water does this, plus it's super gentle, hydrating and will remove all makeup.

A daily moisturiser with SPF 30: this covers off hydration and broad-spectrum sun protection, two things you need every morning. Something basic from the pharmacy like Sunsense Moisturising Face SPF 30+ will do the job.

An antioxidant-rich (vitamins E and C, green tea, etc.) moisturiser without SPF for bed time, or under makeup in the evening. I made one in my skin care range for this exact reason, and unluckily for you I am gauche enough to name drop it right now: Go-To Very Useful Face Cream.

An exfoliating product: I use chemical exfoliants rather than physical face scrubs (go for toners or masks with glycolic or lactic acid in the ingredients), but *look*, as long as your doing some kind of exfoliation 2–3 times a week, I'll award you a credit.

Face wipes for drunk/lazy nights or travel ONLY. Do not make the mistake of thinking using these qualifies as real cleansing. It does not. Also: pricey! Also: The environment!

I hope that helps. Feel free to skip a tutorial today to hit Priceline. Although believe me, when you're paying off your HECS for the next 10 years, you'll wish you'd attended every stinkin' lecture and tutorial on offer, and maybe snuck into a few extras not even on your syllabus, too.

PLUG!

# Q: HOW DO YOU TREAT A VERY (SWEAR WORD) PAINFUL STYLER BURN?

A:

I burn my neck or face with hair stylers or curling tongs far too often. When I explain the wound to other women, they generally nod gravely and point to scars as evidence of their own heat styling mishaps.

And yet, despite the breathtaking frequency of these burns, I always forget what to do. Every time. (Water? Ice? The scales of a green-backed derp fish?)

So, here's what to do! Let's all commit it to memory! And by all, I mean me!

*This is for superficial, first-degree burns only. If the skin blisters and is very sore, red and swollen, go to the doctor: you might have a second-degree burn, sugarplum!*

- Run cold water on the burn, or submerge it in or splash it with cold water, for 10–20 minutes/as long as you can.

- Take some aspirin or Nurofen.

- DON'T USE ICE – it can damage the skin and cause frostbite. Only an IDIOT would use ice. ('Me.')

- DON'T USE ANYTHING OIL-BASED! Including butter! Or oil!

- Next, **either:** Use an antibacterial cream. I use Medihoney Antibacterial Wound Gel – it's soothing and Manuka honey is a terrific healer. **OR:** Apply pure aloe vera gel to the burn to cool it down. Go as strong and pure as you can. I keep some in the fridge for burns now. That says a lot.

- Loosely wrap a dry gauze or non-stick bandage around the burn.

- If blisters appear in following days, do not pop them! Use an antibacterial cream or gel on them to keep clean.

- Don't scratch or pick at the wound. Guaranteed scar if you do.

- Keep applying aloe vera/Medihoney for a few days.

- After 5–6 days, once it has adequately healed (the 'scab' has fallen off), begin scar prevention with a restorative, healing oil like vitamin E, intermixed with Mederma Scar Cream Plus twice a day.

**Disclaimer:** *If a medical person tells you another way to do things, listen. Despite my best attempts to help you treat these stupid burns (and my cute white dress and stethoscope), I'm no nurse, just a klutz who doesn't want you to scar.*

# Q: UM, WHAT IS BALAYAGE?

Balayage is the pastry favoured by the Danish royal family when they get sick of eating Danish pastries.

That's a lie and a terrible one at that. Sorry.

Balayage is actually a hair colouring technique; it means 'to paint'. Hair colour is painted onto the hair, generally in an imperfect, randomly applied way, and rarely directly at the roots, but rather a few inches down, or even just from the mid-lengths to the ends, to create the illusion of natural created-over-time (usually sun-bleached) highlights, rather than the traditional foil highlights.

In short, it's *how* you apply the colour, not *where*.

I love it because I'm incredibly busy ('lazy') and I hate having to get my 'roots' done, so balayage allows me to have some colour and contrast in my hair without very much maintenance at all. I favour some highlights 3–4 shades lighter than my own hair colour, haphazardly placed around my face and all throughout the hair starting a coupla inches from the scalp. (Remember, it's not uniform in application, so there is no visible line of where the hair colour starts and ends – they are sporadic and all-over.)

Balayage is not to be confused with ombré, which infers a two-tone look, with a definite line of colour change.

And as we learned earlier, it's also not a pastry. But if it WAS a pastry, I think it would probably involve custard and I reckon the Danish king and queen would be all over it like white on rice.

# Q: HOW SHOULD I DO MY MAKEUP WHEN I WEAR SPECS?

Here are some suggestions, four eyes. KIDDING. Kidding. I love you and would never call you that. Jess put me up to it. She's such a scallywag, that Jess!

**Conceal the eyes real good.**
The shadow of your frames can make you look like you have dark circles even if you've had nine hours sleep, a week of cold-pressed juices and three facials. So, after you've applied foundation, conceal. First correct any darkness with a yellow- or peachy-toned corrector, depending on your skin tone, then pat on your concealer. Next is illuminator. You might ('will') like to dust around the eyes with loose powder to stop your concealer transferring onto your glasses.

**Define, fill in and shape your brows.**
If you thought brows were important in Non-Spectacle Life, multiply it by four zillion when you enter Spec Life. After all, your brows are now competing with frames for attention. So spend a few minutes filling them in, combing them into place with a spoolie or brow comb, then set them with gel.

**Apply some eye shadow.**
When using and choosing shadow, keep the eyelids fresh, light and bright. Try to avoid dark shades and smoked-up eyes, and super avoid greys or very cool blues. They will most likely wash you out and make you appear tired. Instead, apply soft pinks, lilacs, taupes, bronzes and latte shades over the whole eye socket,

and then use a brown shadow along the socket line and blend it out. Keep the inner corner clean, bright and free of liner – you want as much light in there as possible – and avoid makeup on the lower lash line if you can bear it.

**STOP.**
Pop your frames on and see how it's all looking. Okay. Cute as. Proceed.

**Limit your lashes.**
Maybe don't go nuts with your *Supa Mega Giga Volume Boosting Mascara* when you're wearing glasses, as your lashes will brush against your lenses, and lush lashes are wasted anyway when frames are involved. Instead, curl and then apply a coat of regular/defining mascara.

**Again: STOP.**
Pop your frames on and see how it's all looking. Breathtaking? Okay. Proceed.

**The rest of your face.**
A face in glasses will really come down to a) Frames, b) Brows and c) Lips, so do your blush and bronzer as normal. That said, if you use cream blush and bronzer, be sure to set it with a few dabs of loose powder, or corresponding powder blush and bronzer, to ensure no makeup transfers to your frames. As for lips, and, you know, all makeup in general for everyone, do whatever the dang you like! Go nude, go shiny, go matte, go bright, go BONKERS.

# Q: I'M PREGNANT: WHAT HAPPENS TO MY BEAUTY ROUTINE?

Congratulations! You know, it's funny, I barely remember being pregnant... One day I was having sex, the next I had a tiny baby in my hands!

Also I am a commercial helicopter pilot and can eat 15 hot dogs in 60 seconds.

LIES, ALL LIES.

Pregnancy is a HUGE and TAXING thing on the body. There seem to be 532 rules about what you can and can't do/eat/drink, you get fat ankles, your feet go up a shoe size, the clothing choices suck, your pelvis can fall apart (mine did), everyone comments on your size/your stomach constantly, and if they're not doing that, they're trying to get their paws on your bump or tell you it's definitely a girl. Also you sweat and wee and snore more than you thought one lady body was capable of. Cute!

Of course, it is *all* worth it. Babies are the goddamn best.

When it comes to your beauty routine and pregnancy, there are a few things I recommend, and also some I definitely unrecommend.

**I RECOMMEND:**

• Going as simple and pure as you can with your **skin care**. Skin is an organ. Baby is in your body. Can't hurt to keep things pure while you have a tenant, right?

• Using a rich, hydrating body lotion on your bum, thighs, boobs and tum pretty much as soon as you know you're up duff **to prevent stretch marks**. Yes, they are largely genetic, but it's important to keep the area supple. Continue this until at least 6–8 weeks *after* the birth cos the skin is still moving/changing then. (Fun fact: As long as the dark line down your tummy is still there, you still have pregnancy hormones in your body.)

• The consensus on **dyeing your hair** seems to be a) avoiding it in the first trimester, b) choosing semi-permanent or ammonia-free hair dye, c) skipping a full tint for highlights or balayage from the mid-lengths to the tips so there is no scalp contact, and d) doing what you can to detract from your swollen ankles. (Bright pink?)

• Having your hair cut and coloured and your brows done a week before your due date. (Actually, make it two. Just in case you go early.) Also, **consider keratin smoothing** – I did it so that my hair was wash-and-go while I had a newborn/no sleep/no desire to get out of my PJs for a month.

- **Self-tanning** is safe but go organic for peace of mind. (I love Vita Liberata, Santorini Sun, and EcoTan Winter Skin gradual tanner.)

- Definitely seeing your **dentist** at least once while preggo and absolutely brush, tongue scrape, floss and mouthwash daily, you cute little stinker. One of the sexier pregnancy side effects is inflamed, sore, bleeding gums and manky breath.

- You have a good chance of melasma **(strong hyperpigmentation)** thanks to your preggo hormones: this is tricky to treat because there isn't much a topical solution can do. I settled for strong lactic peels and at-home AHA serums. (See page 38.)

- Enjoy your thick, full hair and plump, juicy, line-free face brought on by pregnancy puffiness. It's bloody gorgeous! *All of you is gorgeous!*

**I UNRECOMMEND:**

- Things with **irritants and toxins**. Skin can be more sensitive when you're preggo, so go easy on it.

- Products with **more than 2% salicylic acid** (found in a lot of acne treatments), also known as BHAs. Small amounts, such as a spot treatment, are fine. If in doubt, switch to AHAs, which will have a similar effect but are deemed safe.

- **Vitamin A, retinol, retinoids**, Retin-A, retinoic acid, retinol palmitate, retinyl palmitate, etc. Not till you've finished breastfeeding.

- **Soy products**, which can aggravate your pigmentation.

- **Oil of bergamot**, for the same reason.

- The DHA in **spray tans** is safe but the inhalation factor can be iffy...I wore a fetching mouth and nose mask

- Go for **physical sunscreen** – zinc oxide- and titanium dioxide-based – over chemical sunscreens.

- If you get **cold sores**, unfortunately you can't take your usual anti-viral tablets: stick to Compeed patches and Lysine.

- Pause your **botox, fillers and teeth whitening** till after you've finished breastfeeding.

- Pause listening to your One Direction album and ask yourself: why am I doing this?

# Q: HOW DO I BEAT A BLIND PIMPLE?

With the technique below, dumdum! It really works! This is good news provided YOU DON'T PICK at it, which you won't. (The bad news is that you *will* pick at it.)

**1** While it's just a painful, red bump, ice it to reduce the swelling. Take an ice cube, and wrap in a tissue. Hold it on the spot for 5 minutes on, 10 minutes off. Three times. Good girl.

**2** When it shows a head, carefully, gently bring the beast up. After a shower (the steam is vital in the drawing-out process), take a clean face cloth or a thick cotton pad and dip it into a sink of as-hot-as-your-skin-can-handle water. Hold this compress on the bump while swearing and kicking the toilet, for as long as possible. Re-dip in the water when it cools down. Do this for five minutes.

**3** Now apply a drawing paste. This is a thick goo made of things like clay, sulfur and zinc oxide. Apply it to the head of the pimple with a cotton tip, and go to bed so it can do its work. You should see an obnoxious whitehead in the morning, (or, as sometimes magically happens, just faint redness, because it's matured the whitehead so fully that it's gone). I love Payot's Pâte Grise for this, and my beloved Drying Lotion by Mario Badescu also works. Old mate Magnoplasm works too, but it's pretty foul.

**4** Time to extract. If it's still red and tender or shiny and taut, no touchy-touchy. Conceal it and repeat the drawing process that night/when possible. But if the whitehead is trying to jump out, then you're ready, Shezzy! Correct extraction begins with either a good steam out, or the hot water compress business on the left. Then wrap half a tissue around each of your index fingers, place a finger each side of the whitehead, then carefully, gently, with NO NAILS DIGGING IN, push down on the sides of it, then kind of roll your fingers upwards to encourage the head to pop out. The idea is to get down deep on the sides, and push the very bottom of the whitehead up and out. Do the same motion from a few different spots to share the pressure (and fun!) around. You should see no blood. There shouldn't even be indentations where you've been pushing: be as gentle as a bee's burp.

5 Once you've popped, bacteria can sneak in, so it's important to seal and heal it right. Apply pressure on the spot to stop potential bleeding, swelling or redness then wipe on a purifying lotion or toner with a cotton pad. Something with salicylic acid, ideally. I like Gernetic's Sebo-Ger, but I'm pretty sure Garnier and Clearasil etc. do them.

6 Now leave it the hell alone for a couple of hours, you rascal. No face cream, no makeup; nothing. (Extractions are best done at night for this reason.) Once the area is flakey and dry, use face oil or pawpaw ointment on the area to encourage healing and scar reduction.

Well, look at this. You avoided a two-week-long pimple-picking nightmare and an unsightly mess on that beautiful face. Congratulations! Your medal is in the post. (You still live at Disneyland, yeah?)

# ESSENTIALS:

Sometimes a lady just wants a quick reference to the beauty products she should have in her...

**HANDBAG:**

1 × concealer OR foundation stick that doubles as concealer

1 × cream blush (with a mirror, if possible)

1 × powder compact or blotting papers if required

1 × black kohl/eyeliner

1 × lipstick of your choice

1 × nude gloss

bobby pins/hair elastics

**Optional:** A Travalo with your favourite fragrance. (Travalos are little aluminium bullets you can pump your own fragrance into. They are magnificent.) Or make your own solid perfume: place some Vaseline into a small tin and spray in your scent, mixing it through the Vaseline as you do. Or just buy a rollerball size of your favesie scent from Sephora.

**MAKEUP KIT:**

1 × foundation

1 × CC or BB cream

1 × concealer

1 × blush (cream and/or powder)

1 × bronzer

1 × black eyeliner (pencil or gel)

1 × neutral eye shadow quad (browns etc)

1 × mascara

1 × nude gloss

1 × red (or pink, orange – up to you)lipstick

1 × fluffy blush brush

1 × thin, angled liner brush

1 × mid-sized eye shadow brush

1 × brow pencil with brush/comb built in

**Optional:** Lash curler, illuminator, corrector (for underneath concealer), loose or regular powder, primer, coloured eye shadow to flatter your eye colour, (see page 96), and all the brushes you see on page 318.

**BATHROOM CUPBOARD:**

1 × broad-spectrum SPF 30 sunscreen
and moisturiser in one

1 × serum treatment product

1 × face oil

1 × face cream with antioxidants

1 × body lotion

1 × body sunscreen

1 × deodorant

1 × facial cleanser

1 × facial exfoliator

1 × purifying/deep-cleansing/chemical
exfoliant mask or peel

1 × hydrating, nourishing, brightening,
firming or radiance mask

500 × fragrances

**Optional:** Self-tanner, gradual tanner, body oil, muslin face cloth, Clarisonic or similar.

**SHOWER:**

1 × body wash

1 × body scrub

1 × shampoo and conditioner

1 × hair mask

1 × razor with inbuilt gel strip

**Optional:** Lavender essential oil and washcloth (chuck the cloth over the drain and drip on a few drops of the oil for an instant day spa steam thingy).

**HAIR DRAWER:**

1 × thermal heat protectant product

1 × (body/volume boosting
or smoothing) mousse

1 × styling cream/texturiser/sea salt spray

1 × dry shampoo

1 × volume dust

1 × hair dryer with nozzle attachment

1 × flexible hairspray

1 × styler brush/Tangle Teezer

1 × cushion/paddle brush

1 × barrel brush

1 × wide-toothed comb for detangling

1 × tailcomb

2638 thin hairbands and 8220
bobby pins

**Optional:** Flat-iron styler, curling tong, frizz serum, straightening/curling balm, root-lift spray.

**CAR:**

1 × lip gloss/balm

1 × mini sunscreen

1 × hand cream with SPF

(And keep them in a dark, hidden, sun-free place, replacing annually.)

**Optional:** Glittery yellow eye shadow, pet rock.

# TOOLS:
## Makeup Brushes

**The Smudger!**
**A.k.a. the 'Push**
**and Wiggle'**
(MAC # 214)

**The Very Accurate**
**Concealer Brush**
(Bobbi Brown)

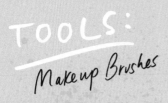
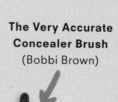
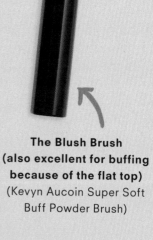
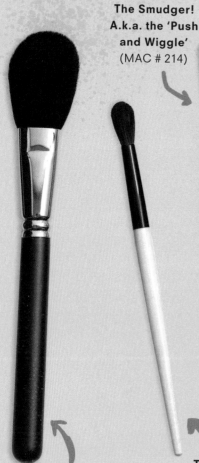

**The Blush Brush**
**(also excellent for buffing**
**because of the flat top)**
(Kevyn Aucoin Super Soft
Buff Powder Brush)

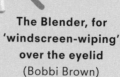

**The Big Loose-**
**Powder and Bronzer**
**Brush** (MAC # 150)

**The Blender, for**
**'windscreen-wiping'**
**over the eyelid**
(Bobbi Brown)

**The Gel/Cream Liner**
**and Inner 'V' Brush**
(MAC # 209)

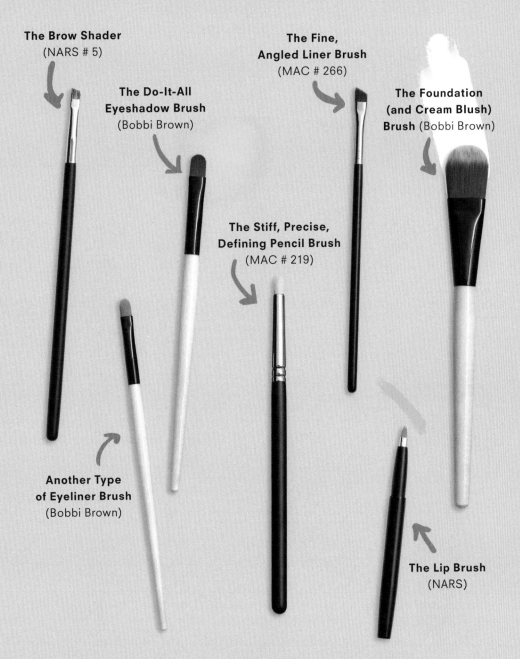

**The Brow Shader**
(NARS # 5)

**The Do-It-All
Eyeshadow Brush**
(Bobbi Brown)

**The Fine,
Angled Liner Brush**
(MAC # 266)

**The Foundation
(and Cream Blush)
Brush** (Bobbi Brown)

**The Stiff, Precise,
Defining Pencil Brush**
(MAC # 219)

**Another Type
of Eyeliner Brush**
(Bobbi Brown)

**The Lip Brush**
(NARS)

# TOOLS:
## Hair Brushes

**Styling Comb**
(for detangling, teasing
and styling)

**The 'Denman'
or Styler Brush**
(for smoothing,
straightening, body
and detangling)

**(Rat) Tailcomb**
(for perfect parts and
wet-hair looks)

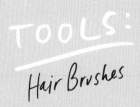
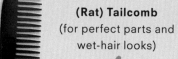
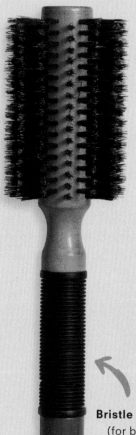
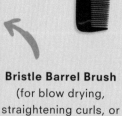
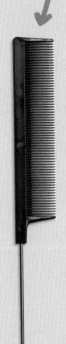
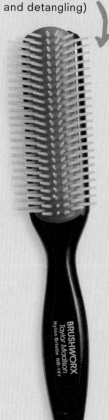

BRUSHWORX
Taylor Madison
Nylon Bristle NB-161

**Bristle Barrel Brush**
(for blow drying,
straightening curls, or
giving a sleek finish)

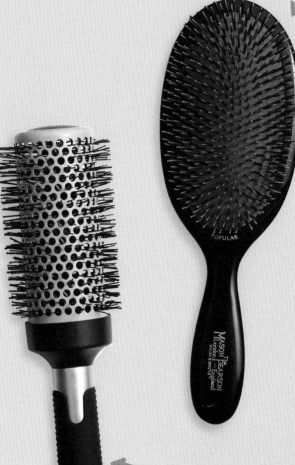

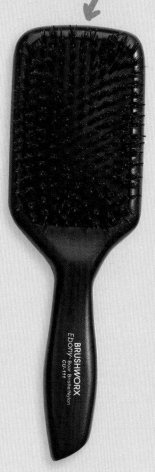

**Cushion Brush**
(for smoothing dry
hair, and on-the-go
grooming)

**Paddle Brush**
(for long hair, smoothing
and straightening)

**Vented Barrel Brush
(tourmaline/ceramic/
thermal/ionic)**
(for fast styling, creating
volume and curl, or sleek,
smooth hair, depending
on barrel size)

# INDEX

# ACKNOWLEDGEMENTS:

## Hey, thanks, you guys!

Thank you Kirsten for sculpting my best 'dinner party' beauty tips into something other than a glamorous mess inside my head. Thank you Allison for your astonishing design, artwork and vision. Thank you to Kim, Nicci, Sally, Cate and all the Penguins who worked so hard on pushing this baby out to sea. (Both times.) Thank you Tara for being awesome, and Mia for giving me my start in beauty at *Cosmo*. (WHY? HOW?!) Thank you to my funny, warm and rascally beauty ed mates for all the fun over the years, and to all the talented hair, skin, nail and makeup pros I've sucked dry for knowledge – I'm immeasurably grateful. Thank you to all the ladybugs who've read my beauty columns, features and blogs over the years – your enthusiasm thrills and delights me. Thank you Meowbert for gazing lazily over my keyboard as I write; thank you Hame for your unwavering support and love; thank you Sonny for being SO, STINKIN, CUTE; and thank you concealer for making me look like an actual person most days.

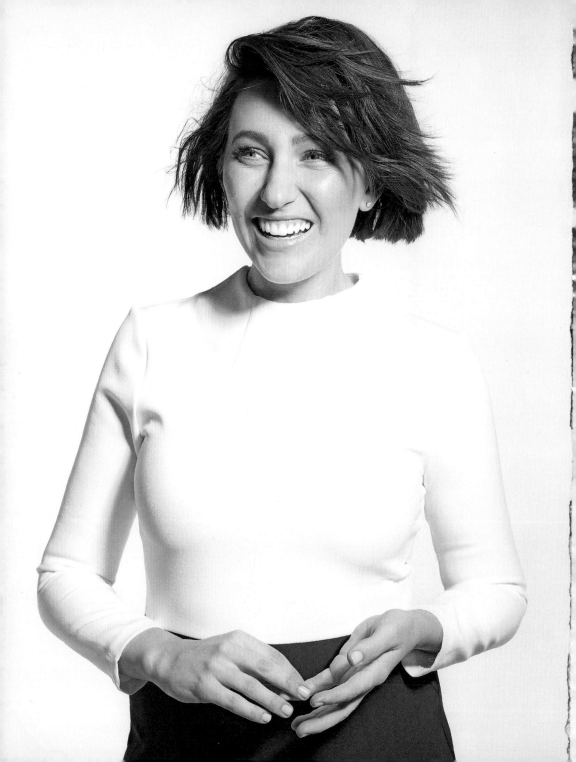

# Zoë Foster Blake

enjoys writing her biography because she gets to write things like 'The literary world was shocked when Foster Blake was controversially awarded the Man Booker Prize for the third time', despite the fact that this is patently untrue.

Things that are true include a decade of online and print journalism writing for titles such as *Cosmopolitan*, *Harper's BAZAAR* and *The Sunday Telegraph*, as well as being the founder of all-natural Australian skin care line Go-To.

Zoë has written four novels: *Air Kisses*, *Playing the Field*, *The Younger Man* and *The Wrong Girl*, and a dating and relationship book, *Textbook Romance*, written in conjunction with Hamish Blake. She wrote the first version of this book, *Amazing Face*, in 2010, but wanted to make an updated-y and better-er and, well, Amazinger version because she cares deeply about her readers being fully informed and up to date. Also there was nothing on TV.

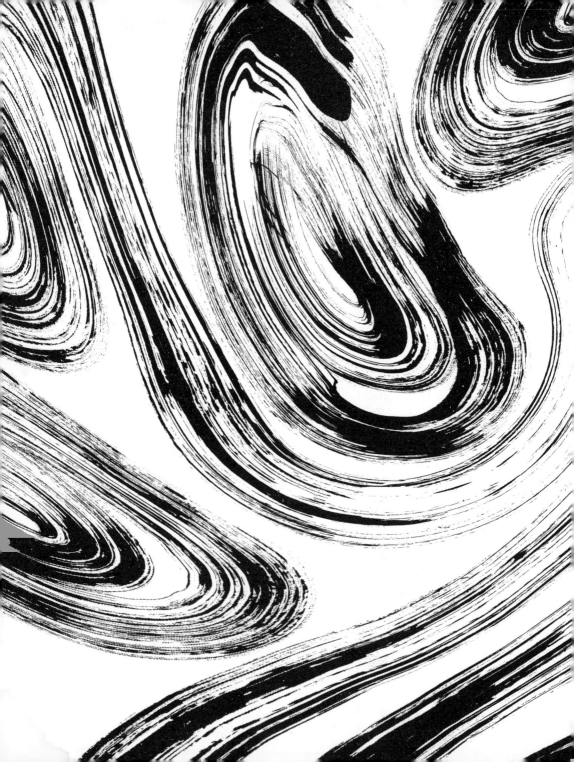